The
Pleasur
Is All
Yours

The Pleasure Is All Yours

RECLAIM YOUR BODY'S BLISS
AND REIGNITE YOUR
PASSION FOR LIFE

Rachel Allyn, PhD

SHAMBHALA

Shambhala Publications, Inc.
2129 13th Street
Boulder, Colorado 80302
www.shambhala.com

Cover art: Sarah Brody
Cover design: Sarah Brody
Interior design: Kate Huber-Parker
Photos on p. 211 © Lisa Venticinque

9 8 7 6 5 4 3 2 1

First Edition
Printed in the United States of America

♻ This edition is printed on acid-free paper that meets the
American National Standards Institute Z39.48 Standard.
♻ Shambhala Publications makes every effort to print on recycled paper.
For more information please visit www.shambhala.com.

Shambhala Publications is distributed worldwide by
Penguin Random House, Inc., and its subsidiaries.

Library of Congress Cataloging-in-Publication Data
Names: Allyn, Rachel, author.
Title: The pleasure is all yours: reclaim your body's bliss and
reignite your passion for life / Rachel Allyn, PhD.
Description: First edition. | Boulder, Colorado: Shambhala, [2021] |
Includes bibliographical references and index.
Identifiers: LCCN 2020048026 | ISBN 9781611808582 (trade paperback)
Subjects: LCSH: Pleasure. | Mind and body.
Classification: LCC BF515.A526 2021 | DDC 152.4/2—dc23
LC record available at https://lccn.loc.gov/2020048026

IN MEMORY OF Marguerite Grahn-Bowman, a pioneering marriage and family therapist and thoughtful mentor to myself and many others, whose kindness and guidance I was so fortunate to receive.

~

Contents

Appendices

Acknowledgments

I feel fortunate to have an expansive community of people who have supported me, whether it be during the early envisioning stages or the manifestation process of this book.

To those who helped plant the seed within me, I'd love to give thanks to: my dad for always being a champion of my education, both indoors and out; to my mother and her mothers, grandma JuJu and grandmother Newton, for modeling writing as a path to healing; to Dr. Ritterman for your guidance in my disparate life stages; to D'ana Baptiste, you and your training were a catalyst in the realization of my dharma; to the leaders of Off the Mat, Into the World—Seane Corn, Hala Khouri, and Suzanne Sterling—your trainings helped activate my passion in action; and to Tim Farnham for your encouragement and heart at the start.

In the later stages of the book I want to extend a heartfelt thank you to my Widjiwagan community, especially the humorous and wise reflections on being a parent in the modern era, as well as Doug Kleemeier who kept me nourished in the final months before my deadline; to my clients, thank you for being my teachers; to the women in my writing group at ModernWell and the colleagues in my consultation groups, I could have never endured the isolation of therapy and writing without you; to my friends who offered to read sections of the book, whether I gave you the opportunity or not, just knowing you were available made a huge difference; to the TEDx Minneapolis team for believing my ideas were worth spreading and coaching me on a talk that helped hone the book; to Katie Silcox and Mariah Rooney, two experts in your fields, thank you for taking the time to share about the important work you each do; and to Lisa Venticinque for the photos and your gorgeous aesthetic, which always captures just what I'm looking for.

A mighty thank you to Andrea Baker for taking on whatever administrative task I threw your way from time to time; you were a lifesaver. To Beth Frankl and Emily Coughlin at Shambhala Publications for your wise feedback that helped add finesse to this project. And heaps of gratitude from deep in my heart to Linda Sparrowe. Linda, you were there with me every step of the way, even when my musings were clunky and un-pleasurable to read! Thank you for believing in me. I truly lucked out working with an editor like you.

CREDITS

"Unwritten," Words and Music by Natasha Bedingfield, Danielle Brisebois, and Wayne Rodrigues. Copyright © 2004 EMI Music Publishing Ltd., EMI Blackwood Music Inc. and WSRJ Music. All Rights on behalf of EMI Music Publishing Ltd. and EMI Blackwood Music Inc. Administered by Sony/ATV Music Publishing LLC, 424 Church Street, Suite 1200, Nashville, TN 37219. International copyright secured. All Rights Reserved. *Reprinted by permission of Hal Leonard LLC.*

"Sexual Healing," Words and Music by Marvin Gaye, Odell Brown, and David Ritz. Copyright © 1982 EMI April Music Inc., EMI Blackwood Music Inc. and Ritz Writes. All Rights Administered by Sony/ATV Music Publishing LLC, 424 Church Street, Suite 1200, Nashville, TN 37219. International Copyright Secured. All Rights Reserved. *Reprinted by permission of Hal Leonard LLC.*

The
Pleasure
Is All
Yours

Pleasure to the People

In a world full of challenging problems, why is pleasure so important? Why are we even talking about it? Because pleasure is our birthright. It keeps us resilient and fosters empathy. And we need to reclaim it now, more than ever, to stay connected to ourselves and to one another. After all, here in the US, we live in a time of fear and angst, bombarded with reports of mass shootings and riots, planetary destruction, viral pandemics, and crises of all kinds as an outgrowth of the unfair systems and structures in place. It can all be too much to bear; so overwhelming that we rage or shut down and disengage. Wanting to escape is completely understandable, but our methods of checking out—drugs and alcohol, food, overspending, screen time, overworking—are too easy to abuse. On top of all that, with everything going on in the world, many of us feel guilty prioritizing our own pleasures.

I get it, but I don't buy it. Paradoxically, as scientific studies confirm, we actually need to engage *more, not less*. We need to find time for pleasure, connection, and intimacy in order to soothe and heal, to strengthen our resolve as well as our nervous systems. We need to feel connected to ourselves and the innate healing capacities of our bodies in order to help us connect with each other.

All of us, every body, wants and deserves pleasure and joy. No matter our gender, sexual orientation, race, class, religion, political leanings, or relationship status, we *all* deserve a life of pleasurable moments that cultivate joy. In a capitalist culture with a history of white-bodied supremacy, access and opportunity to life's pleasures

1

has not been equal. How do we reclaim pleasure for all in a country of disparity? How do we find whole-body health in an unhealthy world? Embodying pleasure is a path to liberation and a form of defiance from the systems that try to limit, judge, or hold us back.

The Pleasure Is All Yours is born of my belief that disconnection from our body, our community, and one another keeps us from accessing kindness and experiencing healthy pleasures. This profound disconnection is at the core of our personal pain and our collective *dis*-ease. To embody pleasure is not frivolous; it is an essential aspect of being human. And being human means more than just going through the motions; it means feeling the full spectrum of emotions, including pleasure and intimacy in all its myriad forms. It means being present to all that is happening in the world—the suffering and the joy—and holding these contradictions within us in order to awaken our ability to care for ourselves and others.

So, how can we wake up?

We start by seeing pleasure as healing. We start with giving ourselves permission to receive it in different forms through a practice called *bodyfulness*, a more physically dynamic version of mindfulness that facilitates ease and delight from within by engaging the natural healing capacity of the body. I believe it holds the key to reawakening our inherent sense of vitality, empathy, and pleasure. Bodyfulness is both a lifestyle and a practical, real-life way to apply new findings in the fields of neuroscience and epigenetics that show how unprocessed emotions live in the body and are healed through the body. It's led to my TEDx talk, workshops, retreats, and articles—and now this book.

Throughout the book I'll share my story of how I became separated from a healthy connection to my own body, and how I found my way back . . . to eventually become a licensed mind-body psychologist with a specialty in relationships and sexual health. I'll also share vignettes of my clients' stories to highlight the ways they transformed through the practices of bodyfulness.

I know from my own experiences and from working with clients for almost two decades that different types of pain are what stand in the way of pleasure. Of course, the contrast between pain and pleasure is sometimes more sharply delineated than other times. An example of my own pleasure-pain contrast occurred in Buenos Aires one lovely spring evening as I walked home after dinner with friends. The temperature was perfect for a stroll, so I blissfully took my time, admiring the architecture, murals, and quaint neighborhood vibe along the way. Suddenly I felt someone brush up against me, grab my phone out of my hand, and take off. Without hesitation, my body's fight-or-flight response kicked into high gear and I chased after the boy, despite the fact that I have *never* been a sprinter and I was wearing sandals. Two blocks and one pulled hamstring later, I gave up. There I was, out of breath, stripped of my handheld portal to the world, not to mention my directions to get home in a new city.

Like the thief who stole more than my cell phone on that sweet spring evening, opposing experiences of pleasure and pain can tangle and butt up against each other. It seems that life is always giving me reminders to not get overly attached to pleasure as a way of avoiding pain. Being fully human means learning to navigate the complexity of both.

Unfortunately, many of my clients were taught that pleasure is self-indulgent and should be avoided or severely reduced—and never actively sought after. Where did they learn that? From a culture that promotes body shaming, violence, and working yourself raw; from their parents, teachers, and religion, as well as the media. They come to me wondering why they feel so detached from their bodies, why they feel blah, why they have no libido, why they are lonely . . . After hearing so many tales of indifference, anxiety, and depression, I wanted to do more than help people feel an absence of crappy. I wanted them to thrive, not merely survive. And the ultimate manifestation of thriving is experiencing pleasure and joy, so I help them with both. And although this book is ultimately about both, I focus primarily on pleasure because it is a building block to joy and because of the way it has been so stigmatized in the US. Joy is undisputed, whereas pleasure is more controversial—it can seduce us and be easier to abuse. They both deserve seats at the head of the table in the feast of your life.

Let's face it—if it were so easy to connect to joy, intimacy, and pleasure, we wouldn't need this book. But we all have our barriers. Day-to-day life can feel lame at times; it can even be brutal. I've found that being an expert in pleasure is also about being an expert in what causes pain. I see how our beliefs and behaviors around emotional pain can translate into physical dis-ease, creating roadblocks to the ways we recover from challenges and receive pleasure.

I've spent countless hours with people intimately discussing their struggles, so I make sure to balance work with my own methods for savoring life, and I want you to do the same. I credit my parents' very different approaches to life for helping me develop my own version of life balance. The '80s T-shirt that best represents my dad's philosophy reads "No pain, no gain"; whereas my mom's is "Don't sweat the small stuff" on the front and "It's all small stuff" on the back (or an image of a cat hanging from a tree branch, reading "Hang in there, baby!"). As a result, I've often felt like E. B. White when he said, "I arise in the morning torn between a desire to improve the world and a desire to enjoy the world. This makes it hard to plan the day."[1] So much of life is about striking a balance. You'll see this reflected in my philosophy and activities around body connection and reclaiming healthy pleasure.

The greatest influence on the exercises in this book comes from yoga history and philosophy, although other embodiment styles and activities are shared here as well. But if you're not a yogi, don't let that scare you off. The word *yoga* can be a bit off-putting; some of my friends and family love yoga and it's a big part of their lives, and others think it's too airy-fairy or falls short as a workout. There's no more powerful way to see the benefits of body connection than to experience the effects firsthand, whether you're on a mat or a mattress. When people move and flow and go inward, there's a visceral aha moment. So if yoga isn't your jam, simply think of these practices as ways to get into your body and get the blood flowing in order to see what comes up and what you can release. Yoga and embodiment practices are just as much a tool to physically soften as they are a way to approach your thoughts and ask yourself important questions, such as *What do I really need right now?* and *How can I best show up in the world?*

BOTTOMS UP

I first conceived of the idea for the book because I was mystified by the ways the US disconnects the mind from the body, and sexual health from human health. Sexual education still barely scratches the surface in most medical school curriculum in the US. What our education lacks, I see the media make up for with misleading and sensationalist headlines, such as "Three Quick Tips for Mind-Blowing Orgasms." If people never learn about the nuances of sexuality, like the fact that it starts with knowing and trusting their body, these gimmicky lists just set them up for failure. As Rumi said, "Maybe you are searching among the branches for what only appears in the roots."[2]

I was also perplexed by how the body was an afterthought in mental health—the *mind*fulness craze being the most recent example—given I'd seen firsthand the improvements that friends, clients, and students made when they engaged and cared for their body. So I went digging, and I couldn't find anything that integrated Western medicine with ancient Eastern wisdom when it came to the integration of body therapies, sexual health, and pleasure—at least not in a way that spoke to the everyday curious person. What I found was either too medical and sterile or too esoteric and mystical. I set out to offer something accessible to every body in everyday language, rather than scientific or metaphysical jargon; a book that was enjoyable to read and helped cultivate body connection and pleasure from the bottom up. Attempting to heal even *one* of these issues—mind/body disconnection as well as pleasure/health disconnection—after centuries of dysfunction is a mighty task, but my hope is you'll see how interdependent they are on the path to more fully awaken in your life.

This book is a road map for bodyful pleasure, an integration of ancient and current theories I greatly respect, applied to our modern times. It's for anyone who wants wisdom without the woo, who values holistic insights that come from current science *and* from ancient practices. Integrating them gives us greater wealth of information, backed by time and science.

People want everlasting happiness, love, and great sex but skip over the work and self-connection to get there, which are so important to cultivating intimacy. This is why I structured the book into three parts. In part one, "A History of Disconnection," I explain why it's hardly surprising that most people from the US don't see pleasure as a birthright or follow the wisdom of their bodies, given the mixed messages handed down throughout US history. This opening section shows us what's possible, gives us the historical and cultural context for how we've strayed so far, and helps us carve out a path toward reclaiming connection to our body, pleasure, and each other.

In part two, "The Body Holds the Key," we dig into ways to feel whole, balanced, and enlivened instead of devalued and disconnected. We hear more and more about mindfulness, which helps us mentally slow down and be intentional. The problem is it can sometimes leave us stuck in our heads, ignoring a profound resource within: the wisdom of the body to keep us grounded and healthy. After all, the language of the body is our mother tongue. This section reunites you with that language to increase body awareness, release stress, and stay awake in your life. I'll explain what *bodyfulness* is and how to make sense of it from a Western medical perspective and the ancient Eastern wisdom traditions. Bridging these worlds gives an expanded understanding of "What exactly is going on in there?" while still leaving room for a little mystery and reverence for the badass vessel you inhabit.

In part three, "Soulful Reconnection," you'll continue to practice listening, understanding, and appreciating your own body, which enhances sharing it with someone else. At this point, you will have been introduced to bodyfulness and have learned what interferes with intimacy. Here you get to put bodyfulness into practice, learning techniques that help you feel at home in your body—even when there's some pain or discomfort—and how to open your heart to others with integrity. After all, the more intimate and appreciative we are with our own selves, the healthier we vibe with someone else.

There's now increasing awareness in the scientific community for the ways stress gets stuck in the body if we don't have ways to dislodge it from the body. Although different therapeutic methods mention that stress blocks pleasure and healthy relationships, they don't focus on how to reclaim it. So much emphasis is on helping people establish emotional safety, leaving pleasure as an afterthought. This book attempts to bridge that gap, recognizing somatic (body-based) theories and methods while also picking up where most methods leave off by specifically addressing the importance of reigniting pleasure and intimacy.

The book is an invitation, not a prescription. It's a recipe for lasting change, not a Band-Aid or a quick fix, as much as I know we all like those! I wrote the chapters in a particular order, and the exercises I've chosen and created are all part of the bodyfulness journey. Engaging in them can help create new body memory, which helps transform the mind. How's that for a one-two pleasure punch?

In this time of increased fatigue, loneliness, and anxiety, *The Pleasure Is All Yours* is a step-by-step guide to help you release the barriers to life's pleasures within you. By owning your right to pleasure, and learning internal methods to embody it, you can feel more vibrant and connected to yourself and others. It's really a book about the power of body connection to cultivate the power of human connection. This is the key to preventing detachment in this rapidly digital, post-pandemic era.

~

Note: I am in support of those who prefer the nonbinary pronouns they/them rather than she/her or he/him. I have tried to distinguish between someone's gender identity, biological sex, and their socialization based on assigned gender. Although there may be times when traditional male and female pronouns are used in the book, this will be primarily for grammatical purposes or to quote research.

PART ONE

~

A History of
Disconnection

~ 1 ~

Your Pleasure Potential

Feel the rain on your skin / No one else can feel it for you /
Only you can let it in / No one else, no one else, can speak
the words on your lips / Drench yourself in words unspoken
/ Live your life with arms wide open / Today is where your
book begins / The rest is still unwritten.

—Natasha Bedingfield

MY FRIEND JJ picked me up for a workout one morning. We've
found it easier to hold ourselves accountable if we have to drive the
other person. Her chariot arrived and as we drove to class she re-
counted a steamy dream from the night before. She was having a
barbecue and the actor Jason Momoa (hunky superhero actor) happened to be there. That's the beauty and randomness of dreams.
Anyway, a flirty energy began developing between them. With come-
hither eyes she beckoned him to help her gather more food from
the kitchen. While they were there, Jason looked her in the eyes and
started to press against her and she . . . ugh . . . she woke up. Annoyed
by this, she somehow—brilliantly—went back to sleep and resumed
the dream. There he was! They picked up where she left off. Talk
about the power of intention. JJ kept part two of the dream to herself,
leaving their escapades to my imagination. He's not exactly my type,
but I wouldn't kick him out of bed.

Our dreams can be dewy wonderlands or complicated mazes.
What happens in our sleeping life is fascinating and misunderstood. As the voice of our subconscious, our dreams are sometimes
connected to our hopes and fears, and sometimes they're pretty

far-fetched. I once dreamed I was on *America's Next Top Model*. Case in point: anything's possible in our dreams, even being a five-foot-four, freckled fortysomething on a modeling show.

I've also gotten lost in all sorts of musings while awake, of course. Everything from imagining what I'll devour after a workout to the way my boo and I will reunite in each other's arms during a warm downpour, Hollywood-style. Engaging in fantasy and daydreaming sparks our imaginations and boosts creativity, compared to when we're lost in thought about tasks or worries.

So let's kick off this book with the power of our imaginations to dream *big*. To dream that we feel completely safe in our bodies because we live in a world free from discrimination due to gender, orientation, race, ethnicity, age, weight, income, and any type of oppressive "othering." Where we have healthy relationships with our bodies, friends, food, creativity, and sexuality. A place where we enjoy presence, play, and pleasure on a regular basis, which gives us the reserves to face challenges and difficult emotions. A world free from shame, guilt, repression, and aggression regarding our feelings, our bodies, and our desires. Envisioning what is possible when we commit to bodyful lives can inspire us to make our dreams a reality.

In my professional life, my dreams focus on my hopes for my clients but also the culture at large. (Of course, I sometimes have less altruistic dreams, such as my TEDx talk going viral—we all have our hustle!) Having only a few hours a month to improve the health of a client feels like a drop in the bucket of a sick culture. Not to mention that many people in the US don't have the means to even see a therapist. My dream recipe for comprehensive health would mean that everyone had health insurance that actually covers medical, dental, and mental health sessions (without the hurdles of high deductibles and denials). People would have time and resources to receive complementary treatments such as massage, acupuncture, and energy work. We would have diverse and enjoyable movement every day, whether it be a walk in the park, basketball with a friend, or a dance class, as well as meditative activities such as stretching and breathing exercises. We would value the health of everyone's mind, body, spirit, and relationships; people over profits.

We would all have work-life balance in the US, instead of just talking about it. Sweden recently instituted a six-hour workday. Imagine what you could do with two extra hours every day (and zoning out on screens wasn't an option)? Speaking of the resource of time, in my fantasy, employees would get *far* more than merely two weeks of vacation. Staff would be encouraged to use all their days off because bosses would recognize how refreshed and focused they were when they returned. No one would feel the need to check their work emails at every stoplight and before they went to bed because the boundary between the office and personal time would be respected.

I can't stop there. As they say, dreams are free; the sky's the limit! Everyone would have the option of a daily siesta to rest and digest. This wouldn't be to catch up from a prior night of tossing and turning about the skyrocketing cost of college for your daughter, the safety of your son from police brutality, or the possibility of being laid off from your job. No one would need a mouthguard at night to prevent their teeth from grinding out their worries. Opportunities for other kinds of restful activities would be encouraged, not judged, leading to more alarm-clock-free mornings, the chance to finally read that book on your nightstand, and the time to replace the dust bunnies in your tub with an Epsom salt bath for your aching muscles.

Kitchens would be stocked with healthy, flavorful foods that you would cook with love and share slowly with others, not scarf down by yourself while standing over the kitchen sink. People would have access to and the money to spend at farmers markets, where they could stock up on brightly colored vegetables instead of hitting up the In-N-Out Burger drive-through. Packaged foods wouldn't contain ingredients no one can pronounce—chemicals like phenylalanine or butylated hydroxyanisole, which the FDA says are safe but we all suspect are toxic.

The cherry on top of my dream sundae would be satisfying, empathetic, meaningful relationships, starting with the relationship with our self. We would appreciate our intentions and unique traits.

Our mistakes would be forgiven and seen as lessons along the way. And we would quite literally feel comfortable with our skin and accept our sun spots and wrinkles rather than attempting to erase them with expensive potions.

There would be a strong sense of belonging to community. We would have time, energy, and opportunities to nurture diverse friendships. Tall fences would be taken down so neighbors could get to know one another and enjoy backyard potlucks, trivia nights, and talent shows. Art, gym, and recess would be priorities in schools so kids could express their creativity and move their bodies rather than be numbed with pharmaceuticals in order to stay put at their desks. Children would have classes on understanding and expressing their emotions, and they would become so fluent in this language that as adults they wouldn't resort to projection, ghosting, or manipulating others to cope with emotional challenges. Everyone would feel encouraged to connect with spirituality in the way that aligned with their beliefs. You do you. Maybe your Guru is you.

We would not only feel safe and at home in our body but also have radical love for our body. From childhood to adulthood, we'd be encouraged to listen to the language of our body and trust and value its messages. Sexual energy within us would be understood as a lifeforce energy that builds connection, creativity, and intimacy—to be enjoyed for the sheer sake of it not just for procreation. Sex would be seen as a way to have fun, feel alive, and bond with another person, with consent and respect at the core. Our bodies, free from fragmentation and commodification, would be on equal footing alongside their bosom buddy, the brain.

This utopia would be a place where all sentient beings are sacred and safe. This would allow everyone to feel the kind of ease that opens them up to luxuriate in life's pleasures on a regular basis—key ingredients to creating states of joy. These ingredients being moments for sensual pleasure—that is, pleasure of the senses—inviting presence, contentment, and satisfaction; playful pleasure that is silly, creative, curious, and non-outcome-oriented; liveliness as pleasure, which is a state of flow, adrenaline, adventure, and purpose; and sexual pleasure that revolves around physical intimacy, eroticism, and desire. This would strengthen our resolve to face challenges and difficult emotions with more finesse.

This idea is similar to tantra, one of the most misunderstood ancient philosophies. It was later popularized by Sting and his wife, Trudie Styler, who revealed they practiced tantric methods so their lovemaking sessions could last all day. Sounds exhausting. As I'll explain more throughout the book, tantra is ultimately about pleasure and joy as basic human rights; this is also at the core of bodyfulness. Just as meditation and mindfulness have become commonplace in modern culture, I dream that a more tantric ethos emerges one bodyful person at a time. And I say to myself, what a wonderful world . . .

DREAM INTERRUPTED

Sadly, there are all sorts of reasons—historical, political, and cultural— why our fantasy isn't our reality, as I will share in the following chapters, not to mention a recent pandemic in which life felt more like a dystopia than a utopia. On the individual level, we've forgotten how to nurture ourselves, or we never learned in the first place. We've disconnected from the very thing that has been with us all along, rooting for our well-being: our body.

So many people are disconnected from their body and what it does for them. For example, many people don't realize that something as basic as changing their breathing patterns can set a ripple effect of calm and nonreactivity within them. Instead, people look *outside* of themselves for a little peace. There is no shortage of distractions around us—screen time, food, drugs and alcohol, shopping, overthinking, overworking, aggression, busyness. They will always be there; my motto is "See them for what they are and avoid being excessive."

Why wouldn't we grasp for soothing distractions in a world full of threat? We have car and house alarms to prevent burglary, yet theft still happens. Bullies lurk not only on the playground but also online and at the office. Don't take your eye off your cocktail; someone might slip you a drug. Hackers Zoombomb video meetings with racist, homophobic, and misogynist rants and images. People now cover their computer cameras for fear of being watched. Computer viruses attack hard drives. And, of course, physical viruses such as the novel coronavirus upend everything we thought was "normal." It will take years to see how we'll recover from this collective trauma. Social distancing and staying at home saved human lives. Time will tell if we become unhuman or more human as we attempt to find ways of coexisting together.

We can't be afraid of inviting in the light because we've been in the shadows. If we live in fear, always waiting for the other shoe to drop and avoiding our aliveness, our life becomes one big attempt to avoid death. We *can* counter our fears by learning and remembering how to insulate ourselves first, because refuge also lies within each of us. This grounding leads us to open up to the possibility that is awaiting with each new day.

INHABITING THE BODY

It's taken me decades to learn how to relish in my aliveness. I haven't always been a full-fledged pleasure expert, although I've been one in the making since the 1970s. Born on the heels of the sexual revolution, I grew up in what psychologists call a "sex-positive" household. My mother never shied away from explaining the names and functions of my reproductive body or talking about what it meant to be intimate. "Sex ed" in my family was no secret and no big deal. Of course, sometimes that was a little embarrassing, like the time in second grade when the teacher asked where babies came from and all the other kids said "Mommy's belly" but not me. Much to my teacher's surprise, I matter-of-factly explained that babies "come from the uterus." Or like the time I offered to help my Grandma JuJu sell her homemade dolls at the state fair, only to discover that some of them were, well, anatomically correct! But I learned that the body was to be celebrated—in all its stages—not hidden. I was taught the truth of my body as a sexual being, which thankfully helped me remain free from much shame or secrecy.

My dad preferred to support all this sex positivity more from the sidelines. But he encouraged me to have a relationship with my body in a different way—through sports. While other kids were getting hooked on Pac-Man, I was drawn to endurance activities, eventually focusing on the grueling sport of cross-country ski racing. Shivering outside in a bodysuit while icicles dangle from your nostrils probably isn't the definition of pleasure for most people, but oddly enough it was for me. The cold, combined with the intensity of the workout, often left me feeling exhilarated and focused.

While I was encouraged from an early age to embrace both the pleasure and the power of my body—as a sexual being on the one hand and an athlete on the other—nevertheless, I was still a female raised in a culture conflicted over sex, pleasure, and the body; a culture that values producing over resting and rewards achievement above all. As a result, it didn't take long before I became trapped in a mind full of unrelenting demands and unrealistic expectations, with little room left for simple pleasures. My relationship to my body became one of punishment and reward and I became disconnected from its need for balance.

But then something changed. I went to a yoga class with my mom, on a whim. The teacher, a seventy-year-old woman named Dottie, dressed in shiny leggings and a leotard, led us through a series of movements as she talked about presence and breathing. Something about her voice and her message touched me and for those ninety minutes at least, I felt free—free from my relentless inner critic and my ever-present to-do list. I signed up. Although I went back to my aggressive, cardio-rich workout regimen (which I still do, but more intentionally), I slowly began to temper it with yoga and other diverse movements, which helped me approach my athletic endeavors—as well as the rest of my life—in a kinder, gentler way. Ultimately this combination helped me discharge the stress from my body and feel more centered.

I had been in talk therapy, which certainly gave me insights but only up to a point. Once I enlisted my body by integrating talk therapy with moving meditations, my overthinking mind got a rest and my patterns changed. I was no longer a thinkaholic. I couldn't just think or explain away the tension. I needed to fully *inhabit* my body instead of *using* it to perform. Research is increasingly supporting this idea, indicating that stress of any kind—whether it's from the day-to-day grind or from a traumatic event— can get stuck in the body unless we figure out how to release it, through crying, raging, sweating, being massaged, running, stretching, tapping, and more.

With a more flexible body came a more flexible mind. I was ready to shift from being critical to being curious; from pushing my body past its limits to embracing its natural limitations. I got certified as a yoga instructor and, at the same time, started to explore all kinds of movement therapies I could incorporate into my work as a psychotherapist. I've been on a journey of self-discovery, sensuality, and body connection ever since. This journey invites me to seek pleasure for the sake of being awake to all aspects of life and, at the same time, insists that I not turn away from difficulty and injustice, which is also an inevitable part of the human experience.

And now I'm happy to be on the journey with you. So, like my friend JJ, let's resume where I left off, to learn how these fantasies could become our reality.

What if . . .

You could be unapologetically yourself?
You could be unapologetic about your body?
You never held back expressing your you-ness?
You validated *all* your emotions?
You felt like *enough*?
You did not fear you were *too much*?
You noticed what needed nurturance within you?
You knew when to self-soothe?
You knew how to self-soothe?
You stayed in relationships that were satisfying?
You left relationships you had outgrown?
You knew when to meditate and had a toolbox of different
    types of meditative activities?

You let yourself have fun?

You could make fun of yourself?

You could buckle down when you needed to work instead of procrastinating?

You balanced socializing with others and time alone for yourself?

You saw time as a gift to be experienced rather than a void to be filled, because you liked being with yourself?

You were able to embrace change without losing your core stability?

You let your body be of service to you—to regulate? To heal? To enjoy? To be kind?

Let my fantasy of whole-person health start to shape *your* blueprint for a life that feels better, brighter, and full of heart. We're all entitled to free ourselves from what *isn't* working and get reacquainted with what *did* work before we lost touch with ourselves. Let's explore how you can make that happen.

Do these simple exercises throughout the book anytime you notice you're overthinking. Start with five big inhalations through your nose as you raise your arms high and five exhalations out your mouth, expanding fully into your abdomen, as you bring your arms back down. Let out a long sigh for the last couple exhalations, softening the jaw and rolling back the shoulders. To get blood moving in your legs, walk to a wall or counter for stability and then do five to ten gentle squats, bending your knees approximately ninety degrees. As you come up to standing, try rising onto your heels a few times to engage your feet and calves. Finish with shaking out one leg at a time.

BIG BLUE SKIES AWAIT

My friend Baron told me he went on a ten-day silent retreat. He explained that he was in an upright, cross-legged seated position for hours on end. It was hard for me to listen to the rest of his story because I couldn't get past the fact that it was *ten. days. still. silent.* My back ached just thinking about it! Not all of us have the time or inclination to make such a commitment. Luckily there are many other bodyful ways to incorporate meditation as a vehicle for transformation in our lives.

I agree that it's important to practice stillness at times to help let go of reactivity and cultivate inner steadiness. That's why the first stage of bodyfulness is *embodied mindfulness*, a practice of slowing down and listening. I also think it's important to recognize how hard it is for most people to bring their fast-paced, on-the-go lives to a screeching halt in order to meditate. Plus, being still and silent in the body can be triggering for some people. This is why Corpse pose comes at the *end* of yoga class. You've moved your body and released the creaking inside; you've let out energy from your cells and tissues and gotten the blood flowing. You've given your body the attention it craves, and this leaves both the mind and body better able to settle in.

I share this because if you keep hearing about the merits of meditation to improve your life and, like me, you struggle with the rules in traditional meditation, I've got your (aching) back. These rules are a reason many people feel like they "fail" at meditating. The pressure to not move at all, even though your body is telling you otherwise, is a rigid turnoff for many. If your back itches, I say scratch your back! Switch the cross of your legs if they're cramping—or sit in a chair!

The more open the definition of meditation, the more inviting it feels, especially for people who are just getting started. I give my clients and students a broad, inviting definition of meditation: anytime you are immersed in your experience, fully embodying the moment, you are meditating. Based on this definition, you can meditate while lying down, walking through your neighborhood with wonder, or chopping vegetables for dinner, as long as you are plugged into your experience without judgment. Likewise, bringing a more open, meditative attitude to movement is crucial to deriving pleasure in the body. And it helps you approach other things you do in your life with more patience. Some meditations are still, slow, and sultry, while others are free and flowing. There are lots of different styles, some I'll suggest in this book, and they're each a vehicle to cultivate more bodyfulness in your daily life.

Over time, presence and kind self-awareness can help lead to *sukha*, which is Sanskrit for "bliss," "sweetness," and "spaciousness." It's like a big, wide-open blue sky. A big-sky definition of self-awareness includes learning how to create space within yourself for *all* your emotions and feelings, not just the warm-fuzzy ones; letting yourself actually be real, which includes feeling *everything*. It means embracing your humanness, knowing that humans are inherently flawed and complicated and marvelous.

Being present is a type of pleasure all its own—the kind that tells you that where you are is where you're meant to be. This emphasis on *being* in the moment is counter to the *doing* and *consuming* capitalism encourages. The irony is the more you practice presence, the more productive you are, if you choose.

I don't want to sugarcoat the meditation process, both the still and moving kinds. The path toward sukha can lead you to your edge as you become more aware of your patterns . . . as you begin to notice how much you think about the past, the future, uncomfortable sensations, and conversations, or even your chipped pedicure. Most of us are experts at living in the past or in the future but not in the present, so it takes real practice to not be busybodies. Throughout the book, try to be open-minded, patient, and spacious like a big blue sky. Given how critical people are with themselves, this can be a radical notion.

Like meditation, bodyfulness isn't about getting somewhere else—it's about embracing and feeling at home in your own fluctuations. It starts with pausing and listening to what's happening in your body with curiosity and acceptance, then engaging in activities that discharge stress from your body so you feel centered and soothed.

Over time this leads to increased mind and body confidence because you have more tools to handle what comes your way. This liberates you to savor more of life in all its wonder and complexities, in all its pleasures.

Learning is all about things being *revealed* to you and later becoming *concealed* from you as you forget. One of my teachers, Coby Kozlowski, said that we are like goldfish who swim around our tanks and when we go by the little plastic castle we think, "Wow, there's a castle!" Then we go on our merry way until we circle back and with newfound awe we think, "Wow, there's a castle!" Fortunately our frontal lobe is bigger than a fish's, so eventually the lessons *do* sink into our mind and body. But we all need reminders and reinforcement. Repetition is the mother of invention. So load up on fish food and be patient as you take some laps around the tank.

Pleasure is your fundamental birthright. You don't have to look to distant lands, buy expensive potions, or find the perfect partner to experience it. You don't have to look to the newest gadget, the pair of jeans that promises to look slimming, or the hot superhero in your dreams. Although you may have forgotten, or you've been too busy to notice, you possess a goddess energy, an inherent vitality, but it's been blocked. Embodied bliss is right there within you, just waiting to be unleashed.

~ 2 ~

Pleasure Is the Measure

Pleasure is a beautiful word. That *s* in the middle,
pronounced like the *z* in azure, a word favored by
lyric poets, gives a little thrill to the mouth.
—*William Safire*

I'VE ALWAYS WANTED to be a surfer chick. Never mind that I was
born and raised smack-dab in the landlocked Midwest. Logically,
rather than growing up a taut, tan surf goddess who could rock a
bikini, I became a competitive skier who rocked long underwear and
wool socks. But both sports share the sense of vitality that comes
from defying gravity. You work your ass off—paddling or poling your
way until you're floating, momentarily feeling the pleasure of utter
aliveness.

In my adult years it became clear that my disposable income
needed to feed my wanderlust as much as my belly. I began traveling to places where I could attempt waves manageable for a newbie.
I also discovered just how fleeting pleasure can be. Case in point,
while surfing on a family trip to the Baja peninsula, the joy I felt was
abruptly shattered when someone else's board crashed into my ribs,
breaking one of them. In an instant, pleasure transformed into shock
and crippling pain, which continued unabated for several weeks. I
came to fear every sneeze, laugh, and cough during my long recovery.

This experience punctuated (pun intended) for me the vicissi-
tudes of pleasure and pain that we all face as humans. Like a surfboard to a rib, such opposing experiences crash up against one
another. This truth bomb reminded me not to get overly attached

chasing one and avoiding the other. I needed to find balance in my relationship with pleasure just as I'd learned to balance on skis and on a board—through trial and error. And what a lifelong practice it's been! But well worth it.

PLEASURE DEFINED

Before we can even get to a place of embracing and balancing pleasure in our lives, it's important to understand its many expressions. I've found that often people have a one-dimensional view of pleasure: it's all about sex. For example, when I mention that I'm a holistic psychologist and *pleasure expert* (yes, this is actually printed on my business cards), I get a variety of responses ranging from confusion to amusement. I even get assumptions about me being an "escort," shall we say. One flirty male stranger at a bar—a close talker with bad breath—exclaimed, "What a great title. I can't believe I didn't think of that!" I sensed this was because he wanted to claim it as his pickup line—and not just with me. Given that the word *pleasure* has been associated primarily with sex, he immediately made assumptions about me and my work. Little did he realize that, first and foremost, I was not in the sex industry nor a sex surrogate—those are quite different fields compared to relationship and sex therapy—and second, no amount of money or beer-goggling would make me hook up with him even if I was.

> Work is the meat of life, pleasure the dessert.
> —B.C. Forbes

Quite the contrary, much of my work is about helping people see that pleasure is more than solely about sex; pleasure is a form of healing, a life-force energy, and the desire for pleasure can inspire our creative juices. I want to educate people on the modern and ancient tools designed to awaken the pleasure that is everyone's innate, essential nature: the pleasure of being alive, the pleasure of having a body, the simple everyday pleasures in life . . . the list could go on and on. The fact that it's so personal is also what makes pleasure so special. Given the many misconceptions about what constitutes pleasure, let's see if I can set the story straight.

Most people define pleasure as an experience they like or love, and so they want it to continue. When we feel pleasure, we naturally open up and lean in, because we want more of the ways it softens us like a warm bath or invigorates us like a cool breeze on a hot day. Pleasure is sensitive to the context in which the sensation is happening—whether you're dealing with a potential lover or trying to extricate yourself from a current one. Had the close talker at the bar been a handsome gentleman who wasn't spitting while he spoke, that moment might have been a pleasurable one.

In addition to the context, there are different types of pleasure. Before we look at them individually, I invite you to think about pleasure as the *dessert of life*. What kind of dessert eater are you? Start by imagining you're out to dinner and the waiter asks if anyone wants dessert. Do you look around, waiting for someone else to initiate ordering? Do you want dessert but hesitate because you think you shouldn't indulge? Do you order dessert because, why not, you deserve it? Or do you pass because it seems too indulgent or perhaps even naughty? Do you order dessert and eat it wholeheartedly but then later regret it and feel guilty? Or are you afraid if you have a couple bites you just won't be able to stop (a dessert throw-down)?

Healthy pleasure is being unapologetic about how much you want dessert, asking for it, tasting it, and knowing when to put the fork down. It's about enjoying and being present for each bite, until your mind, body, and belly feel satisfied. Can you survive without it? Sure you can, but do you want to? To deny yourself the pleasure means missing out on the flavors, textures, and shared experiences of life, which is increasingly the case in our culture.

So, what's the difference between pleasure and joy? Pleasure and happiness? Here's what I think: Pleasure is found in life's little *moments*, initially interpreted by our bodily senses and neurochemistry, which creates mental perception. Both joy and happiness are the sum of many pleasurable threads coming together, longer-lasting feelings based on pleasurable emotions. Joy can be more connected to our spirituality and larger-than-life experiences, whereas happiness can be more connected to our goals, values, and purpose. For all three—pleasure, joy, and happiness—our perception is also influenced by what our minds *believe* is going to feel good or not, based on past associations.

The moments of pleasure sprinkled throughout life are the soil and fertilizer for the more lasting feelings of joy and happiness to bloom. All of which helps us stay resilient. But when pleasure is overdone or abused it doesn't really make us happy or joyful at all. It's a nuanced skill to find balance with pleasure because life will always present challenges, and temptations to escape them will always exist.

More so than joy or happiness, pleasure is associated with reward, a treat you deserve, that cherry on top. Sometimes people even self-inflict discomfort to justify receiving the pleasure of no longer feeling pain on the other side, such as running a marathon, which opens them up to a longer lasting state of joy. There can also be gratifying pleasures that are done to avoid suffering, such as the pleasurable gratification of avoiding a *negative consequence*—for example, going to the dentist to avoid cavities.

Everyday moments can be bursts of pleasure if you're intentional about finding them. Like any embodied experience, receiving pleasure requires slowing down, savoring, and staying out of the over-analyzing mind. It requires an absence of being self-conscious and guarded. Being easily embarrassed and overly concerned about what others think about you blocks your experience of pleasure—whether you're dancing, playing a practical joke, delighting in an orange, or having an orgasm. So in addition to this bodily aspect, there is the element of giving yourself permission to *be you*, and to *receive* what feels good, simply because you're a human being. This stands in opposition to the dour and modest influences many of us have been raised with. As I'll explain, letting yourself receive pleasure is an indication of how emotionally and physically safe you feel and how much you believe you are worth it—just because you are you.

Beyond your own experience, a healthy relationship with pleasure recognizes that pleasure is a natural and fundamental *human* experience, part of the natural flow of life's energy. Pleasure is always attempting to contact us. When we limit or deny our pleasure, we are essentially limiting or denying life. Embracing the uncertainty of life is not always easy, but the alternative is a much harder way to survive.

So pleasure is a bodily experience beginning at the visceral, neurochemical, and sensory levels. Want to feel more joyful? Get acquainted with your pleasures. Want more moments of pleasure? Be in your body. I believe the most joyful and compassionate people consistently practice being connected to their body. Your body is also the canvas that guides you to know what pleasure is and is not for you. As you go through the book, keep asking yourself these questions: "Does this feel pleasurable? How do I know this, based on my body's response?" "How might this contribute to my feeling of joy or connection with someone else?"

Make a list of answers for each of the following questions: "What brings me pleasure?" and "What does *not* bring me pleasure?"

Although most people equate pleasure with good sex and creative bedroom play, there really are four kinds of pleasure—sensual, playful, lively, and erotic/sexual—that overlap in myriad ways. Some professionals also suggest that benevolent, altruistic behavior is a type of pleasure. I definitely agree, as long as no one confuses it with overly self-sacrificing behavior at the expense of their own needs, as many women have been socialized to believe is their only role. To them I would say you can't measure your *right* to pleasure based only on the happiness you bring to others. We need to be considerate and respectful of others on our pleasure path of course, but your pleasure should not be solely dependent on someone else. Although I touch upon altruistic pleasure throughout the book, I've chosen to focus on the other four types because they're more frequently discounted or reduced only to sex.

SENSUAL PLEASURE

Slowing down, listening, and igniting satisfying sensations is what sensual pleasure is all about. I love how I feel when I smell the heady scent of jasmine, for example, or experience the sun on my face after a long gray spell. I love petting the soft fur of my orange cat or belting out my favorite song as I head on down the road. Sensual pleasure is all about paying attention to the textures, sights, sounds, smells, and tastes that come in through your senses and responding to them viscerally, which is at the emotional level rather than the intellectual level.

> And forget not that the earth delights to feel your bare feet and the winds long to play with your hair.
>
> —*Kahlil Gibran*

As much as the senses are the pathway to pleasure, they can also be the pathway to aversion, as I discovered, along with a plane full of passengers when Charlie, a ten-pound Chihuahua, made his presence known on a long-distance flight. Charlie's owner apparently decided having him in a carrier would be too confining, and her *Vogue* magazine was too engrossing to pay attention to his meanderings. I watched him as he walked down the aisle, sniffing around the cabin. From where I sat, I got a front-row view of Charlie spreading his legs and taking a crap in the middle of the walkway. The fumes spread like wildfire. Everyone on the plane gasped, barely able to breathe. There was no escaping our olfactory senses.

Whether we're experiencing pleasure or pain, it all starts at the senses, which we'll explore more in chapter 10. Why? Because when we are connected to our sense perception, we are smack-dab in the present moment; we are connected to our aliveness. Unfortunately, much of the time we are sleepwalking through life because we are in our head, detached from our sensual selves, and this prevents us from having agency to minimize the discomfort or maximize the enjoyment of our senses.

One of the body's most basic, primal languages is that of the senses informing our perceptions and emotions, which leads to our feelings, thoughts, and behaviors. Sensuality helps us become more receptive; we have to notice sensations in our body in order to notice our emotions and interpret their messages accurately. Competitive athletes might train themselves to push past their sense perception of physical pain and focus on controlling their mental perception. But if we are routinely cut off from our senses, skipping over them and perceiving solely through the mind, "we cannot heal what we cannot feel."[1] Our sensual connection informs our perception of ourselves, which is important to building overall body awareness and self-awareness. Somatic therapist Manuela Mischke-Reeds explains, "The more you can listen to your sensations, the more your perception gets trained to see without bias. Sensations are the raw data."[2] When connected to our sensual self, we are tuned in and tuned outward to the world around us more clearly.

Noticing your unbiased sensations—and really listening to what they have to tell you—encourages a curious mind of self-inquiry. Note there's a big difference between listening and judging. Listening to the cues of your own body helps you understand its language and inform you on ways to keep in balance and thrive. Coming into your body, breath, and senses also helps you get away from the limited story lines and drama of your overthinking mind, replacing them with the actual reality of your experience in the moment. This leaves you aware of something you certainly have more influence over.

Ask yourself, "What are my barriers to noticing sensations? Is it busyness? Past trauma? Overwhelm?" It's not unusual to discover that when you feel pain, you disconnect from your body by trying to shut off your senses, freezing your muscles, or spacing out.

Being sensual is tricky. Even when you're on board with the idea, there can be so much noise in the way. With everything coming at you from the outside world, your senses can get flooded by competing sounds, images, and smells, and it can be downright overwhelming. Similarly, your own mental landscape can be just as hard to tolerate when you're stuck in a racing mind of obligations and criticisms. None of these scenarios put you in a place of ease. Being in your sensations is about slowing down and getting quiet from the inner and outer noise. As the saying goes, the less you speak, the more you can hear.

Sensual experiences, especially ones that are pleasurable, help open us up to an expanded, unbiased type of perception about ourselves in the world. Understanding the role of our senses means you can have more clarity and make better choices with the tool of sense perception in your toolbox. Keep that field of perception open by finding as many pleasant sensual experiences as you can, inviting presence, ease, contentment, and satisfaction! Practice this by closing your eyes when you take your first bites of food; listening to music and letting yourself release sound through singing and even sighing; using essential oils on your pillow, body, or with a diffuser; or doing what my cat does best—finding a ray of sun and lying in it belly up. Reunite with the little sensual moments around you. Notice areas of ease in your body as well as areas of tension. Bring loving touch to the areas of tension, giving yourself a neck or foot massage. All of this helps you start to feel more at home in your body.

PLAYFUL PLEASURE

One of my best friends teaches pottery. After years of figuring I might suck at working on a pottery wheel, I finally gave it a try. I wanted to make a coffee mug that looked like a coffee mug, but every time I tried, the clay would spin off the wheel or flop over into a pile of mush. Midway through one of the first few classes, I became so

> It is a happy talent to know how to play.
> —Ralph Waldo Emerson

frustrated that I decided to leave early. But instead, for whatever reason, I gave it one more time, resolving to embrace whatever flopping the clay might do. I thought, "Who cares about making a perfect mug. I have plenty of perfect mugs." As soon as I made the decision to let go, something clicked. I put my self-doubt on hold and simply had fun with the process. I started to feel an intuitive understanding for the rhythm of the wheel. Not that I made a perfect mug (or even anything that remotely resembled one), but I did end up with some awkward-looking objects that work as jewelry or pet dishes to show for my efforts.

Playful pleasure is about being creative, curious, silly, and non-outcome-oriented. When I told my friend that I help people have more balanced pleasure and play in their lives, he said, "Oh, you mean like foreplay?" I chuckled and explained that yes, sexual foreplay can be playfully pleasurable but that playfulness outside of sex is also important to our well-being (and a building block to great foreplay). After all, adults make playdates for their kids all the time but not for themselves. As early twentieth-century psychoanalyst Carl Jung wrote, "The creation of something new is not accomplished by the intellect but by the play instinct."[3]

Where to begin? There are all types of play, according to Stuart Brown, the founder of the National Institute for Play. He explains in his TED talk that there is *body play*, which releases your spontaneous urge to defy gravity; *object play*, which gives rise to better problem-solving skills; *exploration and imaginative play*, which helps enhance your creativity; *social play*, critical to your sense of belonging; and *rough-and-tumble play*, which gives you room to explore chaos and emotional regulation. Clearly play is purposeful, and playful stimulation can hit on all our synapses. When was the last time you connected to your play instinct?

What's unique about play is that it can arouse your nervous system, but because it's arousal without overt danger, you can learn to associate that arousal with something pleasurable rather than fearful. If you feel nervous as you embark on the unknown and it turns out to be enjoyable, your physical and mental memory then pairs future new activities with the possibility of pleasure. My experience in the pottery class helped me gain confidence in my ability to grow from attempting something unfamiliar. Just like when I bungee jumped in Zimbabwe at Victoria Falls. With a stunning view and body memory that had experienced enough new playful experiences to keep me courageous,

I was much less fazed by the fact that they attached my ankles to the bungee cord with something that looked as flimsy as dental floss!

So not only does play provide an opportunity to *learn* from new experiences, the pleasure you might take from those experiences can override your trepidation around the risk of something new in the future. This dynamic between play and pleasure can also help you face the risk of being intimate and emotionally vulnerable with someone else. And here we are full circle back to foreplay.

How do you allow yourself to enjoy and revel in the kind of play that leads to pleasurable and reparative experiences? By learning to awaken your creative self. With my clients and students, I like to offer reminders rather than imperatives. It's about *remembering* how it felt to be in your body and in the creative part of your mind when you were a kid—before you were told *not* to be so expressive. Once, while I was at a beach patio in Costa Rica, a DJ was playing to a small crowd of adult tourists scattered about at their tables. A family arrived with a little boy who immediately ran toward the DJ and began clapping and twirling around. We adults were like driftwood scattered about, practically sticks in the mud, while this boy was a wise little octopus, his limbs like tentacles moving freely and happily. You still have this instinctual and playful pull to music within you; it's just buried under years of deconditioning.

Creativity gives us balance by using a different part of the brain. Imagination, intuition, art, music awareness, holistic thought, and creativity are all controlled by the right hemisphere of the brain. The left hemisphere governs more analytic thought, rationality, logic, science, math, and numbers. If you miss that creative side of yourself, remember that creativity is a skill you can cultivate, just like anything else. Sure, you could do some of the more obvious creative activities such as taking a painting, pottery, or poetry class. But you can also enhance your creativity by any of the following:

- Taking dance classes in which you're using each side of your body in different ways, balancing both hemispheres of your brain.

- Having idle time in which you're not *doing* something productive but rather relaxing and daydreaming, letting your imagination wander.
- Experimenting with how you dress and style your hair and makeup.
- Playing around with how you decorate your home and office.
- Building a sandcastle at the beach or making a scavenger hunt.

Having a little more play in your life could be the jumpstart you need, especially if you're struggling with apathy. Cultivating a curious mind allows you to learn new things and see situations from different angles and perspectives. It challenges the "crisis of imagination" that happens when people settle into routine and complacency. You may find it liberating to mix things up—just for the sake of variety. Discover different ways of expressing yourself and notice how it feels to let go of any preconceived *outcome* when you do—like a final dance performance, art exhibit, or taking a class where you get a letter grade. Let go of your version of making that perfect ceramic mug! Too often people focus exclusively on an end goal and don't let themselves enjoy the creative learning process along the way.

Brainstorm all the ways you used to play as a kid. Think indoors, outdoors, at school or home, and during all different seasons. Notice what comes up inside your body as you jog these memories, paying attention to the emotions that arise. Add the ways you've noticed other kids around you be playful and even the ways you've observed pets engage in play.

LIVELY PLEASURE

Lively pleasure is connected to adrenaline, rhythm, adventure, and immersion. It's a state of flow, born of intrigue and focus, where you operate from a deeper inner layer. This type of pleasure stems from activities where time practically stands still—like how surfing has typically been for me (although I may need to switch to something less intense like golf one of these years). For many, myself included, nature is the perfect playground for fostering this sense of aliveness.

> Mountains and oceans teach us in ways that weekend workshops and podcasts never will.
> —Jamie Wheal,
> Flow Genome Project

Given that the fastest-growing migration is to the city and the indoors, you may have to really look for it these days.

Lively pleasure can flourish in physical endeavors and adventure travel but also your livelihood when you're absorbed in a professional project. Examples could be a surgeon's unshakable laser-like focus while operating (which is certainly how I'd want them to be if I were on the table) or a writer completely absorbed as their words unfold a story. This is when concentration is sharp and sustained, moments when "time slows down. Self vanishes. Action and awareness merge," explains Steven Kotler, an expert on the concept of flow. "With our sense of self out of the way, we are liberated from doubt and insecurity."[4] That sweet spot between boredom and anxiety when we have just the right amount of adrenaline is described as the *flow channel*. Different parts of you align because it's *go* time!

When I lived in Utah, mountain biking and all types of skiing were the main ways I felt alive. Of course, it helped that it was all right outside my front door. When I moved to Minnesota, I had a real adjustment period. I felt an ache in my heart for the mountains and the outdoors. But eventually I adapted and grew to love discovering the vast bike commuting trails within the city.

A few summers ago, there were reports of bikers on a main city path getting mugged at night. Friends suggested I avoid riding my bike home from work after dark. But my evening ride was a meaningful ritual, and I couldn't bear to give it up. It was a moment to feel free and live with a little abandon. With the efforts of the day behind me, I would hop on my mountain bike, jump on and off curbs or little trails, just like I did back in my Utah days. I would make my way along the lakes, breathing in the nighttime air, feeling the wind in my hair, and seeing the lights reflected in the stillness of the water.

Given the crimes on the bikeway, my decision to keep biking reminded me of the Take Back the Night movement. More than the title of a Justin Timberlake song, Take Back the Night began in the 1970s as a way to protest all forms of sexual, relationship, and domestic violence.

Perhaps my nighttime biking escapade was my way of taking back the night. I'm not going to give up something I love just because it could be risky. Heck, anytime we get out of bed we take a risk. We also take a risk if we choose to stay under the covers. I'm definitely more cautious now. I have brighter lights on my bike and I always wear my helmet, despite my hair wanting nothing more than to blow in the wind.

Sometimes, on purpose and with intention, I don't do what is safest and it makes me feel alive. It's okay to want to live on the edge a little. There are plenty of ways for us all to break free from our doldrums, to liberate ourselves and have fun or feel passionately absorbed—if we give ourselves permission. These activities help reawaken something inside of us and provide an invigorating pleasure all their own. Having an adventurous attitude that is open to possibility and letting yourself be a bit vulnerable is key. Here are some ways to get started:

- Brainstorm a list of all the places you dream of traveling to. Let go of any excuses, such as "I don't have the money" or "I don't have anyone to travel with," and delve into fantasy. Then start researching new places to explore within your own region, whether it be as earthly as an arboretum or as celestial as a planetarium.
- When were you last immersed in a work project? Think of a time you were "in the zone," engaged in a state of energized focus or passion. Let that inform where your flow channel could turn on (it might be in attempting something more challenging at work).

- You don't have to suddenly become a skydiver or storm chaser to feel adrenaline. You can begin closer to home. Take a kickboxing, spin, HIIT (high intensity interval training), or martial arts class, even if this is a little outside of your comfort zone (heck, *especially* if this is outside of your comfort zone—that's the point). The sweatier the better. Ignore any self-critical voices that imply you're not doing it "right" and instead embody the fiercest version of yourself.

Depending on your disposition, this type of pleasure may require a real pep talk as you weigh the level of calculated risk in each activity. Or you may find it second nature to chase after adrenaline but you're simply out of practice because your life obligations have gotten in the way. Whatever your temperament or life circumstance, it's about creating—and seizing—the opportunity to plunge into this type of pleasure.

SEXUAL AND EROTIC PLEASURE

Sexual and erotic pleasure revolves around intimacy, desire, eroticism, and sex. Consider that foreplay doesn't just begin in the bedroom. It exists in every aspect of your life. First, a quick distinction: any animal can have sex (the perfunctory *behavior*), but humans have capacity for eroticism (the romantic or sexual *experience* and energy you share with another person or evoked from art or literature). Sexual desire is physical, while erotic desire is soulful. Our sex drive is a biological force (to procreate), but it's also driven by our existential fear of being alone. Whereas eroticism is more than just a behavior, more than just momentary companionship from someone.

Sexual healing is good for me / Makes me feel so fine, it's such a rush / Helps to relieve the mind, and it's good for us. —Marvin Gaye

If you're not able to embrace the types of nonsexual pleasure we've just discussed, then chances are your sexual pleasure will be lackluster or unsatisfying, and you may not feel erotic much at all.

Being out of touch with your senses (the language of your body), playfulness (creativity), and aliveness (adventure and vulnerability) probably means you're merely going through the motions in bed or maybe rejecting sex completely. (Granted, it might also have something to do with your options for a partner.) Our right to healthy sexuality is tied to our body connection and our right to feel and want. Fortunately, the other three types of pleasure are certainly building blocks to help reclaim those rights.

A paper published by the Planned Parenthood Federation of America with the Society for the Scientific Study of Sexuality listed scientific evidence on the health benefits of sexual expression. They found that sexual activity—whether it be with a partner or as self-pleasuring—is associated with increased longevity, immunity, pain management, self-esteem, and a reduction in stress.[5] I've known people who credit masturbation for helping them with everything from headaches to writer's block.

The truth is you *are* a sexual being. You come from sexual beings—your parents and their parents and on through the ages. Beyond merely perfunctory efforts at procreation, sexual pleasure is also your fundamental birthright and makes for a much more intimate experience. Yet many people have conflicted feelings around giving and receiving pleasure to themselves and in their sexual relationships. Some find pleasure a lavish, gluttonous indulgence; others fear they will become too attached to pleasure and not have the boundaries to create a balance between work and pleasure, so they avoid it. Both can translate to a guilty conscience that blocks sexual pleasure. Technically, guilt is the belief that you did something wrong, that you went against your values. It's defined as a feeling of responsibility or remorse for some offense, crime, or wrongdoing. In which case, why would guilt be merited within a consensual and pleasant sexual experience? Real or imagined, guilt certainly squashes any possibility of carnal pleasures. Of course, it can rear its ugly head no matter what kind of pleasure you yield to—not just sexual.

This type of pleasure is for many the most likely to trigger stressful feelings about the vagaries of wanting it or doing it "right." Know that it's completely okay to have times in your life when sex and eroticism are or aren't priorities, which I'll talk more about in later chapters. When the time is right, try these pleasure-producing suggestions (and be patient with yourself . . . don't expect to suddenly become the poster child for all things sultry):

- Start to connect with sexual and erotic pleasure by imagining any celebrity crushes you have. Ask yourself, "What is it about them I desire?" List out some characteristics. Next, ask yourself, "What does that bring out within *me*?"
- Pay attention to artwork, literature, drama, photography, or film that stirs up erotic feelings for you. Notice where in your body you feel that energy.
- Imagine a time you felt infatuation about someone. Was it lust and, if so, where did you feel that in your body?
- Imagine a time you felt romantic love for someone. What activities did you want to engage in with them?
- Imagine a time you felt emotional attachment for someone. What did you long to create with that person into the future? It's just fine (and quite common) that all three of these are the same person! The point is to familiarize yourself with the evolution and ebb and flow of sexual and erotic pleasure (*and* how it's about more than just intercourse).

We'll flesh out how to cultivate this type of pleasure in all sorts of ways in our final chapters, but for now let yourself start to envision what healthy sexual pleasure means to you.

THE MIDDLE PATH

Have I been able to persuade you yet that pleasure is a raison d'être—an incentive for showing up and navigating this complicated life? I hope so, but I need to offer this caveat: practice living from the "middle path" between avoiding pleasure on one side and overindulging on the other.

For many people, pleasure elicits their inner Goldilocks—too much and they feel lavish, sinful even; too little and they either feel resentful, dismal, and deprived, or, conversely, overly proud of the self-control they've exerted. I know people who won't grant themselves pleasure unless they've toiled sufficiently, gone above and beyond, exerted blood, sweat, and tears . . . and even then, only allow themselves a morsel, lest they "overindulge." Or perhaps they maintain so much willpower for so long that their body finally bursts and they go on a pleasure bender!

There are also people who cannot tolerate discomfort and instead race to pleasure and sensation-seeking as an avoidance method—a way to anesthetize themselves. This is not a viable strategy. We can't escape the fundamental reality that life can be downright hard and heartbreaking at times. It's all a cycle. We accept that the sun phases out for the moon, that day gives way to night, and that feeling awake surrenders to sleepiness. We understand what happiness is because we've been sad, and so it is with pain and pleasure. We can't have one without the other. Learn to ride the inevitable waves of discomfort and realize it can teach you something, even if it's just appreciation for the ease on the other side.

The relationship therapist Esther Perel, born and raised in Europe, argues that America has a national ethos to struggle around self-control. "People in the United States are massively hypocritical. Everything is exaggerated here, everything is world-famous, the portions are gigantic. It's all about excess and control," she says. "In Belgium you don't sit and eat a meal and talk about all the things you shouldn't be eating because it's bad for you. Being bad is a pleasure."[6] How do we navigate this paradox—a culture with messages to live large and go for the gusto (whether it be eating a double bacon cheeseburger or driving a Hummer) and, at the same time, messages to buckle down, self-sacrifice, and not call attention to ourselves?

Most people *don't* navigate it. They get overly attached to one mode of relating to pleasure or the other: either chasing it and indulging as often as possible or rejecting it and depriving themselves completely. When I work with clients who always chase feeling good, I help them learn to tolerate uncomfortable emotions in their body instead of using pleasure as a way to avoid them; to understand that some adversity is integral to the human experience. For those who withhold, I help them break free from the illusion of control and see what positives can come from loosening their grip.

Both extremes happen in a culture that doesn't teach us to honor the natural, instinctual parts of ourselves or to find the pleasure balance that's so important. Instead, most people rely on trial and error, ricocheting between restraint on the one hand and excess on the other. Some are able to dance this dance better than others.

Bodyfulness is aimed at helping you awaken to your full range of emotions, to all you can receive, feel, and create in the world, and to find your balance. It's about immersing yourself in every experience, recognizing that everything is temporary and savoring it all the more. If you learn that you're capable of riding the ups and downs of your emotional experience, you won't fear the possible darkness. You'll be able to let yourself live with more fervor because you trust that you can pick yourself back up again if things fall apart.

Of course, the very idea that things could "fall apart" keeps many of us from feeling joyful—from embracing pleasure—so that we won't have anything to lose and won't get hurt later on. Brené Brown calls this "foreboding joy." She says that "our actual experiences of joy— those intense feelings of deep spiritual connection and pleasure— seize us in a very vulnerable way. When something good happens, our immediate thought is that we'd better not let ourselves truly feel it, because if we really love something we could lose it. So we shut down our ability to completely enjoy it so that we can also shut down our capacity for feeling loss."[7] Our problem with pleasure isn't just about being socialized to repress it but also our fear of loss and getting hurt. To embrace healthy pleasure, we need to tolerate ambiguity and vulnerability, and find strength and resolve within the capacity of our body.

I'll talk about the different types of stress and trauma that can live in our body and prevent us from pleasure in part two. For now I'll say that spending all our time staving off what we think of as negative possibilities or certainties is called *negative motivation*. If we work so hard to avoid possible problems, how can we have energy for things that are life-affirming?

Take the Pleasure-Measure Quiz in the appendix to see where you fall on the pleasure spectrum. You'll receive a score with corresponding suggestions for how to best connect to balanced pleasure in your life.

PLEASURE IN PARADISE

I get to witness people melt into the first three types of pleasure most often—and with the least amount of resistance—when I host my yearly weeklong retreats. As a kid who loved summer camp well into my high school years (and who still considers my old campmates close friends), it's not surprising that I now lead retreats. I see them as essentially adult summer camps. And grown-ups need these getaways as much as kids do.

I marvel at the transformation that takes place in a mere eight days. How does this happen so quickly? First, by removing people from their home environments with all the dishes, laundry, and yard work. (Plus, it doesn't hurt that my retreats are in tropical destinations.) This creates space and freedom from the busy "monkey mind" that's constantly analyzing and planning. Away from their to-do lists, retreat goers can settle into their bodies with the daily yoga classes each morning and meditation classes each evening, all outside in a beautiful setting. Nature and sunshine obviously play a role, and people get to spend their free time hiking, swimming, boating, horseback riding, surfing, and more. Since sometimes less is more, people also have plenty of free time to rest, whether it be napping in a hammock or reading a book by the pool. And let's not forget all the fresh, healthy, flavorful food. Pleasure in so many forms!

Top all that off with the fact that they often make new friends and strengthen the relationships with the people they came with. Several women whom I met thirty years ago at summer camp are still my cherished friends. Three of them helped me get four feet of fly tape out of my hair (dead flies and all) by lathering my long locks with butter. (How do you *not* notice fly tape hanging from a "biffy"—what we called little wooden outdoor bathrooms in the North woods—and walk backward into it? By being distracted by how gross the compostable toilet is.) How does this relate to pleasure? You don't get these types of bonding moments while vacuuming at home or typing in your cubicle. You sometimes need to remove yourself from life's monotony and embark on an adventure.

People go on retreats for all different reasons—to recover from divorce, the loss of a parent, escape work stress, or celebrate a birthday. They arrive in all types of formations—mothers and daughters, romantic couples, old friends, and people who are traveling solo and wanting to take time to reflect. No matter the arrangement, I witness people connecting to their innate sense of pleasure on these trips not because I'm *teaching* them so much as I'm *reminding* them. As a facilitator I'm reminding them how to reconnect to parts of themselves that have become buried. I see them reunite to the part of themselves that isn't so self-conscious or restrained. The environment and connection to their bodies open them up to remember how to *feel* as opposed to *think*, to *be* as opposed to *do*, to *release* as opposed to *repress*, which sometimes means letting go with tears to make space for laughter.

You don't necessarily have to travel to distant lands to feel more sensual, playful, lively, or erotically connected to yourself or your lover. You can infuse more *pure vida* at home by traveling inward to the intelligence of your body, connecting with your right to pleasure and learning the internal methods to embody it. Then you too can feel more vibrant and connected to sacred intimacy within yourself and others (it will just take longer than an eight-day retreat). So strip off those wool socks and hop on that surfboard—because you never know where riding the wave of pleasure will take you.

Just like most parents do for their kids, make a playdate for you. Here are tips to help ensure that it happens:

- Pick roughly the same day/time each week and try to reserve at least one hour for yourself. Let's face it, when we get into a routine, it's more likely to happen. Consider this time nonnegotiable and sacred.
- Review the suggestions at the end of each pleasure category (sensual, play, lively, erotic/sexual) and choose ones to engage in during your allotted playdate time. Altruistic pleasures are wonderful as well, giving you pleasure from the sheer act of seeing others happy.
- Cultivate some creativity within these suggestions by making them your own—combine the ideas or see how they can inspire you to find new ways to engage with nature, art, a novel activity, or people in your community.
- Practice keeping this playdate time non-outcome-oriented; the less "productive" the better.

~ 3 ~

Expression, Not Repression

Religion says: The body is a sin.
Science says: The body is a machine.
Advertising says: The body is a business.
The body says: The body is a fiesta.

—Eduardo Galeano

TO RECLAIM OUR RIGHT to pleasure and create a world that values
intimacy and play, we need to figure out how we lost all that in the
first place. We need to understand why it's so hard for Americans
to connect with our bodies, to enjoy being in our bodies and have
healthy physical intimacy with others. Our uptight, stuck-in-our-
heads, pleasure-shaming culture could be our first clue. It certainly
has been centuries in the making. By exploring the broader historical
and cultural context for how we got this way, we can see why a much-
needed social and cultural sea change is long overdue. We can see
how conventional medicine, by separating the mind from the body,
has contributed to separating us from our body's wisdom; how fear-
based messages about the "primitive" body and about the dangers
of sex beyond procreation led to an atmosphere in which people
became cut off from pleasure and intimacy.

Pleasure shaming is alive and well, as I was recently reminded. My
morning airwaves are typically set to my trusty NPR station. One day
I bumped my clock radio, accidentally nudging the dial. I suddenly
heard the voice of a preacher in the middle of a story about pleasure
as "the path of the devil." To paraphrase Neil Armstrong, it was one
small change of the radio dial and one giant change of life philosophy.

45

I listened as the preacher carried on about how pleasure was a wolf in sheep's clothing and that we'd be damned to hell if we indulged in it. He warned of the many temptations surrounding us and how we must brace against a culture oozing with sinful distractions, taking us off course from a chaste life. He explained that the enemy exists all around us, but also within our own dirty cravings, so we must exert total willpower. Although the preacher never said the word *sex* (heavens no), it was clear that the most sinful of all pleasures was carnal lust leading to hanky-panky (unless, of course, it was for procreation purposes within a heterosexual marriage). Scratch that itch and you'll go to hell. The takeaway: your desire to enjoy life and feel pleasure, especially pleasures connected to your body, has been disparaged as wanton cravings and giving into temptation.

I was taken aback. It was too early in my morning for a shame sandwich. Was this really happening on the radio in the year 2020 or was this Throwback Thursday? I felt like I had time-traveled, entering the town from the movie *Footloose*, where the community wasn't allowed any fun pleasures such as dancing (until the kids revolted). But these messages weren't relics of the past. They were present day. It reminded me that pleasure-shaming viewpoints remain just a short radio dial (and presidential candidacy) away. And it became apparent to me, yet again, that we must reclaim our right to pleasure. The sooner we figure out how it got lost in the first place, the quicker we can put the pieces back together to feel whole.

MIND-BODY SPLIT

Being disconnected from our bodies and shamed away from pleasure have been centuries in the making. Black and brown bodies were commodified while white bodies became particularly severed from their emotions and feelings. Why? The history of slavery. In a panel discussion called "Wellness Beyond Whiteness," the Reverend angel Kyodo williams expressed, "Black, brown, and indigenous folks were dismembered while white folks were disembodied; they

> Pleasure's a sin, and sometimes sin's a pleasure.
> —*Lord Byron*

became disembodied because how else does a body tolerate that kind of viciousness, how else does a body tolerate the witnessing of that kind of decimation. . . . How else does that happen to a body whose natural inclination is to feel care and connection?" This was handed down through the generations and literally cut people off and dulled them from their own feeling state. This severing is what made them disembodied. To be so removed from compassion and dignity toward others that you are not even connected to what it means to be human is more than just illness, it is what Reverend williams calls "massive sociopathy."

In addition to racism, religion has shamed people away from their bodies and emotions. In 2017, the psychologist Tina Schermer Sellers wrote a book on the origins of sexual shame in American culture, titled *Sex, God, and the Conservative Church.* In it, she explains that Christianity and early religious dogma created a strong distinction between the mind and body, a *mind-body split,* which is the notion that our body and our soul are two different things. Our bodies, according to the early church fathers (and, yes, they were all men) remain stuck in the evils of the physical world, while our souls transcend our base desires—and transcend they must. Giving in to physical urges—the worst being sexual temptation—means you are weak and immoral. If you abstain or take vows of chastity you are seen as even purer. These are the people who make it to heaven. Everyone else? Tainted sinners.

Based on these beliefs, it's not surprising that Christianity in early America became known for spreading fear-based messages about pleasure, the body, and intimacy. The Puritans led the charge when they arrived from England in the sixteenth and seventeenth centuries, becoming poster children for all things grave and repressed. They were only one of many religious groups such as the Quakers, Dunkers, and the Seekers that held strict moralistic rules back then. These groups believed to varying degrees that engaging in pleasures of the flesh took time and attention away from one's duties to God. All forms of pleasure beyond just sexual—dancing, singing, playing cards, celebrating holidays, and so many other types—became demonized because they distracted from living a pious life. Quite the uptight bunch. Our human pull toward pleasure may be primal and natural, but our religious conditioning has covered it in shame and judgment, making anything pleasurable synonymous with sin.

Although shame about the body and sexual desires exists in many subcultures, it has reached epidemic levels among religious communities to this day. Sadly, these tend to be groups in which people confess their desires to the very people who scold and shame them, hoping (usually in vain) to receive support, only to be scolded and shamed all over again. Conversion therapy is an example. It's a program aimed at suppressing or completely changing the sexual orientation and gender identity of someone who has identified as homosexual or bisexual. Through counseling, interventions, and ministry, the programs try to make the person identify as heterosexual. Incidentally, the founder of one of the biggest conversion therapy organizations in the country recently came out as gay, expressing his own feelings of shame and remorse for hurting people with this movement. Yet another closeted conservative leader externalizing his internal gay conflict.

WHAT WE RESIST, PERSISTS

Emotional and physical needs within you don't simply go away because the church (or the media or a parent) has decided you shouldn't have them. Chronic repression is not the solution—it actually creates *more* problems for people. The longer you ignore your basic human needs, the more they demand resolution. Ignore your hunger and your stomach will growl louder. Try to bypass sleep with caffeine and you'll fall asleep behind the wheel instead. Ignore your libido and you'll develop any number of mental and physical challenges that will present themselves later.

This is because *what we resist, persists.* Resist your emotional desire for sensual soothing, laughter, or physical touch and your mind-body system will take that unmet need and shut down some part of itself in an unhealthy way of coping (ulcers, headaches, lock jaw, etc.), which I'll explain more thoroughly in chapters 6 and 7. Or you'll more covertly find ways to get those needs met (having an affair, hiding pornography, engaging in online chat groups). We can be very resourceful at not owning up to our afflictions. The problem is, when the buildup of repression in our body eventually presents its bill, we feel more than just sticker shock.

Everyone deserves to learn about their body and the full range of human sexuality in a factual, nonjudgmental way. They also deserve to learn about the ways pleasure can be *non*sexual and show up in many forms. This empowers each person to make their own decisions about integrating their sensual and sexual self with their spiritual self. In an article in *Psychology Today*, the psychologist David Ley writes, "It is only when a person accepts their sexuality as an aspect of themselves, and not something that is external to them, that a person can truly begin to heal from shame. Then, and only then, can they evaluate their sexuality from a position that supports their own health, in a way that promotes healthy sexual values, in their lives, relationships, and even their soul."[1] For some it will take radical acceptance to embrace that as a human being it is natural and normal to experience pleasure in their body in different ways.

The truth of your body can set you free. But you need to be adequately educated to even know what that truth is. Among the sixteen sexual rights that the World Health Organization created is the right to accurate information. Yet the United States remain a country that debates what should be included in sexual health education—giving inaccurate sexual health information or no information at all. As I'll discuss more in chapter 4, much of this information is meant to induce fear about sex, totally leaving out how the body works and the possibility for pleasure and intimacy.

MIND OVER MATTER

Western medicine has also played a role in separating the mind and body while dissing pleasure. Conventional medicine (as opposed to holistic or functional medicine) claimed the mind was superior, pristine; the body, in contrast, was seen as primitive and not to be trusted.

The medical establishment saw the body as something to be fixed when it "broke down" and became ill, refusing to accept that the body can *prevent* illness with the right behaviors. In his seminal book *Coming to Our Senses: Body and Spirit in the Hidden History of the West,* the social critic Morris Berman writes that we have had a systematic "devaluing of the body itself as a source of identity and authoritative knowledge about our direct, lived experience of the world."[2] Until recently, our thoughts were considered totally separate from sensory perception in the body. Western medicine believed that thoughts led to emotions, which then caused a bodily response; the mind and brain were the conductor, it was a top-down approach. These days, with more research and advances in neuroscience, medicine and psychology have begun to understand the bidirectional nature of emotions, actions, and thoughts. Aspects of the body's response system, such as the nervous system and enteric (gut) brain, are increasingly recognized as having more influence over our mind and behaviors.

Traditional psychology in the United States also focused on mastering the mind as the method of transformation and healing. Here again the rational mind reigned supreme, whereas the body was crude with its wanton urges. The slogan was "Train your mind to tame your body." This is still a prevalent message today. The four dominant strategies we have historically used to deal with difficult thoughts and feelings have been (in chronological order): (1) push it away, ignore, pretend; (2) believe it, let it become the story; (3) notice the thought and replace it with your new thought (cognitive behavioral therapy [CBT] approach); and (4) notice the thought and label it "just a thought" and let the associated feeling come and go without criticism (the mindfulness approach). The fourth one at least is a self-compassionate approach, but the role of the body is barely an after*thought* (pun intended).

Women's bodies and sensuality were especially ignored, misunderstood, and shamed. The origins of modern psychology stem from older white men, most famously Sigmund Freud, who first claimed women's sexual problems were all due to penis envy. He later revised his theories and acknowledged that women's unmet sexual fantasies could lead to physical and emotional distress. He labeled it *hysteria*, meaning a defect in the womb, which became akin to a woman being crazy. Women to this day are called hysterical for expressing strong emotions and opinions.

WE ARE ALL JUST MACHINES

The Industrial Revolution in the late seventeenth and early eighteenth centuries saw the body as a machine to be controlled, not a process or experience possessing capacity to will and create. As the agricultural economy transitioned to mass production with new machines and new sources of power, it was all about efficiency and productivity. This era brought us the philosopher René Descartes and his famous declaration, "I think, therefore I am." Rationality was worshipped; mind over matter. Here again the body was considered savage and listening to its desires a hindrance to productivity that would prevent moving industrial civilization forward. Faster, cheaper, and more was the name of the game. "From the time that we humans began to sharpen our wits we began to dull our senses," Christine Caldwell writes in her book *Bodyfulness*. "The marginalization of the body has such a long and cross-cultural history that we barely notice or care that the oppression of our bodily selves is constant, insidious, and potentially devastating."[3] We barely notice until the body raises its voice with lethargy, panic attacks, insomnia, or other diseases and illnesses—which is pretty counter to all that productivity they were after. And certainly not very pleasurable. This is because we are not robots; we are sensate beings.

These waves in US history—religious, medical, industrial, cultural—each had their agenda, whether it be a ticket to heaven, a long life, more money, or supremacy, respectively. Yet they all attempted to maintain order by controlling humans—either through repression, shame, censoring, or propaganda, all of which remain tools for social control to this day. All four movements believed that they could get people to curb their impulses. A common thread between them was the emphasis on the *rational* mind as a way to control people's *emotional* body. The rise and fall of emotions were seen as chaotic and distracting rather than something to learn and grow from. Emotions such as contentment and stoicism were considered good because they are simple and stable. Emotions such as rage and grief were considered bad because they are intense and not linear—and they could lead people to rebel. Those in power were not down for that.

Repressive religions, the rise of capitalism, and conventional medicine, within the unfair structures related to race and class laid the foundation for a beleaguered, disembodied US culture. The cultures and subcultures of bodylessness continues to this day. As I'll share in chapter 5, our history has morphed Americans into detached, disembodied robots from centuries of bullshit rules on what's an acceptable way to be an emotional, embodied human. No wonder so many of us are short-circuiting.

You don't have to get swept up in this public shaming; there are ways to protest these old messages and return to the lively, expansive emotional creature that you are. Practice the movement exercises listed in the appendix to remind yourself that you are more than just a brain attached to a physical frame.

Censorship around sexual health is alive and well and I recently experienced it firsthand. In March of 2020, I partnered with the organization Allbodies to give an online presentation to their subscribers on ways to communicate about pleasure. Allbodies first became popular on Instagram under the name "Cycles and Sex," providing education on all things related to the female reproductive body and sexual health. Their straightforward and provocative approach, which aims to help women understand their bodies, initially gave them a strong following. Then they started to notice they weren't getting as many "likes" or followers and some pictures had been taken down. They soon discovered that Instagram had decided to hide or remove accounts with the word *sex* or *pleasure* in their title or content. So they changed their name. I had also noticed my own Instagram account was hidden and censored when my handle was @pleasure_expert.

It's hard to spread my message of "Pleasure to the People" when it's hidden from the people.

New information can also be suppressed if it threatens to overturn the old guard. Anything pioneering can face pushback. This has been happening with body-based therapy methods that try to integrate with Western medicine. The United States is a medicalized culture that's been invested in throwing a pill or a potion at people to cure what ails them. In 2016, the US pharmaceutical market was valued at $446 billion.[4] No wonder it sees holistic medicine, which says the body is a resource for healing and illness prevention, as a threat to the status quo.

I ran into opposition after giving my TEDx talk in February of 2019 on bodyfulness as a way to reclaim healthy pleasures. The video wasn't uploaded to TED's YouTube channel until months after everyone else who presented that day. For it to be released at all, I had to send them pages of empirical studies supporting the use of somatic methods. Even then it came with this disclaimer: "While some viewers might find advice provided in this talk to be helpful as a complementary approach, please do not look to this talk for medical advice." Apparently I'm that groundbreaking! I get that we live in a litigious society and organizations want to protect their liability but don't radicalize a commonsense approach to health and well-being just because the word *body* is in it. This begs the question, what will it take for the scientific community to legitimize somatic practices such as bodyfulness, the way they have mindfulness over the last couple decades?

Apparently the answer is more research, given that we value science over the subjective experience of the individual. The challenge is to bridge the gap between the felt experience of the individual with the objective, quantifying nature of science. The potency of our lived experience can get muddled as we attempt to articulate what we experience in our private inner world to those on the outside, especially the analytical realm of science. Our culture views "real science" as coming from laboratories and not people's lives. While I work on the front lines with my clients, I'm happy to see that there *is* a growing body of research on the impact of somatic methods such as yoga, dance, and other types of intentional movement improving people's mental and physical health. Advances in neuroscience—such as our ability to measure the structure and function of the brain—are giving credibility to what monks and yogis knew five thousand years ago (not that they needed scientific proof to validate their inner knowing).

The current philosophy in holistic medicine to treat the totality of the person—their body, mind, consciousness, spirit, and soul—actually dates back to Hippocrates in the fourth century B.C.E. Although we've strayed from its premise for centuries, it appears that holism is making a comeback. An increasing number of US medical schools and think tanks now have departments devoted to mind-body research and treatment and to sexual health across the life span. More research is helping mind-body medicine to escape its negative association with being *alternative* medicine, as terms such as *functional medicine, complementary medicine,* and *integrative medicine* become more accepted.[5]

INEFFABLE

Scientific research is based on quantifying and measuring things. But when it comes to a sensual moment in your body, the chemistry you have with a new lover, or the way you feel after a swim, measuring these visceral experiences—or even trying to put them into words—can't really do them justice. Which is part of what makes these moments so magical.

The *New York Times* bestselling author Michael Pollan wrote a book about psychedelics called *How to Change Your Mind.* As part of his research for writing the book, he experimented with "magic mushrooms" and later shared just how challenging it was to put his experience into words, even as someone who so skillfully describes things for a living. Our history has left us clueless and without the language to intimately understand and describe our felt experience. We don't have a distinct word to express a state of being deeply alive, present, and aware in the body, probably because we can't name something that we don't know how to feel or has been actively marginalized. These experiences are ineffable. It's become easier for people to remain numb, detached, or separated from their felt experiences, given we don't have a vocabulary to describe it. People also fear judgment for speaking out loud, from their heart, about their more tender experiences. So many people are walking around looking for their glasses, not able to see that they're already on their head.

OTHER WORLDVIEWS

According to the World Association for Sexual Health, the United States is one of the most repressed countries in the world when it comes to enjoying pleasure—on par with the Vatican and predominantly Muslim countries.

We have to look beyond US borders to get a more enlightened and practical view of our right to feel good. Healthy conversations around pleasure can be found in many other cultures. In the Netherlands, children are encouraged to be spontaneous throughout their lives and see playfulness and expression as more important than obedience.[6] Singapore and Korea devote extra time in school to the pleasures of creativity and inventive thinking. In the Dominican Republic, children are taught to dance bachata, a style similar to salsa, and continue throughout adulthood. A US friend living there said they "sing like it's their last song and dance like it's their last dance." In France, they discourage rushing meals; an hour lunch break is considered the minimum.[7] In Brazil, the concept of *tudo*, or "everything," refers to the world of erotic experiences and pleasures.[8] Switzerland's and Germany's progressive sex ed programs encouraging pleasure have been linked to their high rates of satisfying sex.[9] Organizations such as the South and Southeast Asian Resource Centre on Sexuality are talking about pleasure as an integral part of healthy sex. Even in Turkey—a country certainly not known for its support of women's sexual pleasure—a program emphasizing sexual pleasure as a woman's human right was created in the 1990s.

These organizations and governments throughout the world were able to recognize expression and pleasure as a fundamental component of overall human health. In the United States, we overlook the topic or actively refuse to talk about it, even in a medical context. As recently as 2011, the word *pleasure* was removed from the US surgeon general's sexual health doctrine after it had initially been included in 2001. These hot-button issues rise and fall with the politics of the time, too often regressing. The more things change, the more they stay the same. That's why we need to start the revolution within ourselves.

A PATH BACK HOME

The natural state of pleasure and sexuality, essential to all humans, is not the problem; the dysfunction (in the form of shame and sexual violence) that has emerged from the fear-based messages we've received is. This historical disconnection from our bodies and the shaming of our emotional desires are why a balanced relationship with pleasure seems to elude us.

> **Our bodies know that they belong; it is our minds that make our lives so homeless.**
> —*John O'Donahue*

These long-held convictions have left quite an impression on us, threatening us away from pleasures of all kinds. No wonder we feel more anxiety and disconnection than ever—we've been trained to be hypervigilant against any semblance of carnal enjoyment and not to trust ourselves. So many people are conflicted, feeling either that they don't deserve pleasure when it's available to them, or they must grab as much as they can, whenever they can—moderation be damned.

Being able to appreciate all our emotions and trust in our ability to learn from them and regulate them is the ultimate personal liberation. Pleasure, like all our emotions, is inherently awesome, but it needs to be in balance for us to make the most of it. Looking for pleasure from other people or external things, without knowing how to feel soothed and balanced within yourself first, can lead to dependency on things outside yourself. It's natural to want something enjoyable to continue, but if you're grasping for it in ways that mess with the rest of your life, then it becomes an addiction. Buddhist philosophy sees attachment as one of the main sources of human suffering. Being too attached to things—being dependent or addicted—creates a never-ending chase for more of something that was temporary from the get-go.

Think of the freedom you could have if you trusted your body intelligence and the ability to practice balanced, intentional "hedonism" (the pursuit of pleasure). In Sweden they call balance *lagom*, defined as "just right," "in balance," and "perfect-simple." Hopefully someday we can strike this balance and shift the cultural view of sensual, playful, lively, and erotic pleasures from something bad or shameful to something normal, healthy, and worthy of cultivating and even celebrating.

Learn to enjoy pleasure without creating more suffering by overly attaching to it. You *can* train yourself to find balance with what you crave. Adopting an intentional approach to pleasure is about choosing accountability and consciousness over avoidance, denial, and numbing. It comes from listening to your inner limits and set points within your mind-body systems and then having ways to discern and find balance inside yourself, which you can learn to do with bodyfulness.

BODY AS WILDERNESS

Making our way back to bodily wholeness requires quite a paradigm shift. The psychologist Tara Brach uses the analogy of the wilderness to describe the landscape of the body. Our history's emphasis on the body as out of control, the site of trouble, and a place of unbridled emotion is akin to the way Western civilization has viewed the wilderness. Just as we've dominated the wilderness for our self-interests, slowly killing the planet, we've tried to dominate the body. Even the concept of *dominating* stems from a masculine, divisive approach rather than a feminine and nurturing one.

What if we reclaimed the idea of the wilderness of the body, seeing it not as unruly and harmful but as natural, wise, unfettered, and connected to the rhythm and order of the universe? Brach says that it is only if we're awake right here in this living body can we connect to what we cherish in life. We can't think our way to freedom, to liberation. Contemplation and reflection are useful, but it is outside of the realm of thoughts that we can really come home.[10] The wilderness is meant to be wild and free, just as our bodies are meant to be wild and free. When we love and listen to the body's needs, responding with some TLC, we can embrace and embody the animals that we are.

To heal we must feel. All people, all bodies, all feelings. Those that arise within us and those that we see in others empathically. We start by cultivating our capacity to be embodied, be body-full, and be in our emotions around care and connection, which is our true nature. This is what the Reverend angel Kyodo williams says is more than just a social justice issue; it's a human rights issue.

~ 4 ~

Boys Will Be Boys

We have been raised to fear the yes within
ourselves, our deepest cravings.

—Audre Lorde

AS A CHILD OF THE '80S, my nostalgia tells me it was the best era of music, movies, and television. Classics such as *The Cosby Show* (who knew?) and *The Facts of Life* taught me so much about, well, the facts of life. I especially loved the shows that involved singing and dancing, such as *Fame*, where the students would break into choreographed dances in the lunchroom.

I memorized all the words to the Marlo Thomas and Friends *Free to Be You and Me* record as well as *Grease* and later *Flashdance* (even though my sister and I were forbidden to see it because it was rated R). I became an expert at making mixtapes, handcrafting the right tunes for the right vibe. Singing and dancing were natural and joyful ways to express myself back then.

Although my body danced without a care, my mind wrestled with the lyrics. Cyndi Lauper told me that "girls just want to have fun," but other messages told me only certain kinds of fun were okay—not the kind involving boys or a brazen attitude. Madonna described being "like a virgin touched for the very first time," while other messages implied a virgin is what I'd better be when I get married. Cyndi and Madonna—as well as Mrs. Garrett and Mr. Huxtable—were part of the village that raised me, within a world of mixed messages about what it meant to be living in a body assigned female and daring to derive pleasure from it.

Fortunately, I was raised in a household that had a good balance of gender-fluid, body-positive messages. I knew I was different when in eighth grade I told my best friend that my mom had thrown me a "party" to celebrate getting my first period. She couldn't imagine such a thing in her house—her family never discussed these sorts of "incidents." (This didn't exactly work in her favor; she wasn't even sure which hole her tampon was supposed to go in.)

Given that no one else in my class seemed to have as open conversations about the reproductive body with their families, I thought there was something odd about mine. I was well into my adulthood before I could own that all this knowledge wasn't a sign I was creepy but rather that I was informed at an appropriate age about essential aspects of myself—things as concrete as anatomical names of the body. I wasn't creepy, I was just *different* from other kids around me because I knew the truth about my body and sexuality rather than relying on the media or the girl next door to help me make sense of it all.

My experience certainly wasn't the norm for most of my friends and many of my cisgendered, white, middle-class clients. I know from listening to them that most parents weren't comfortable talking with their children about the body unless it was about how to control and manage it. And they certainly didn't learn age-appropriate ways to invite pleasure into their bodies, *especially* pleasure associated with sexuality. Instead, they heard made-up words such as *hoo-haa* for vagina or *pee-pee* for penis. The actual anatomical names for the body and the ways the body can aid in both resiliency and pleasure were left out. This leads to such confusion for kids, and even worse, to body shame.

More typically, information was delivered in the manner my client Sara described. Around the age of ten, she was reading in the living room and became chilled, so she threw a blanket over herself, crossed her legs, and warmed her hands between her thighs for a moment. Her mother walked in and saw the shuffling of Sara's hands under the blanket and assumed she was fondling herself. Her mother yelled at Sara to stop what she was doing immediately and *never* touch herself there again. And then—*poof*—her mom was gone;

the one-sided conversation over, no questions asked, no explanations given. What a mind trip for this poor ten-year-old.

I could see how indelible this moment was in Sara's memory as she shared it. Her sense of self was forever changed with the message that a whole region of her body was not only off limits but repulsive. As an adult, she came to me because she still struggled to like her body and because she hadn't felt interest in touch from her husband for much of their relationship. Sara's experience is hardly unique. I'm willing to bet most people have an early life story related to shame around their body and pleasure that they've carried into adulthood. If touch and expression are shut down when you're a kid, of course they will be hard to embody with your partner as an adult.

Our earliest imprints can have lasting effects on our ability to feel worthy of pleasure or to be able to let down our guard and experience it. Sara's experience is a powerful example of how early messages about the body can have harsh, long-lasting effects, especially when those messages include how wrong it is to receive pleasure and comfort from your body (even if it's just using your thighs to warm your hands). The absence of frank, educational, nonshaming conversations about the human body, gender, intimacy, and healthy pleasures has left people confused at best and traumatized at worst.

That tug-of-war I felt between my natural human curiosities and the societal messages I received telling me they were wrong remains true for many kids today. From day one, American kids receive messages about their body and intimacy from parents, teachers, religion, and media. But what trickles down to an impressionable kid is a mere fragment of the whole story, much like being that last person in a game of telephone.

Sex is a biological term, whereas *gender* is a social construct. We all grow up with messages about what it means to be a "boy" or a "girl," and we learn acceptable forms of self-expression for our gender (body language, appearance, hobbies, and how to be in relationships) as it intersects with our race and class. As Sarah Rich explains in The *Atlantic*, "A baby's sex creates a starting point on a cultural road map that the whole family and community can use to direct the child towards defining who they are, and who they are not."[1] Think of the fanfare and "gender coding" for babies before they're even born, like the new trend of gender-reveal parties, a more dramatic version of a baby shower. Although there might be greater awareness today for gender being on a spectrum, consumer culture pushes distinct gender categories more than ever.[2] By making separate versions of the same toy—one pink and one blue—companies can make more money. The same is true for clothes, snack food, and school supplies—all things that have a big influence on the developing identity of a child.

The shaping of gender identity may start more innocently with colors and toys, but over time these "rules" to conform can put people into lifelong boxes that confine them. This influences how kids understand their bodies as tactile and sexual beings, and how they understand their emotions as emotional beings. For some, it leads to a lack of acceptance of their bodies and an inability to communicate how they feel, which prevents meaningful connections with people. For others, it can also lead to deep shame and feeling at war with their body.

Thinking back to your own childhood, what were some of the messages you were told about your body regarding your assigned gender? Were you shamed for your choice of clothing, hair, or hobbies? Were you a girl who wanted to play football with the boys during recess and got teased? Were you a boy who wanted to play dress-up and your parents refused?

If you were raised male, you might have heard messages encouraging you to be tough all the time: "Be a man." "Grow some balls." "Don't be a sissy."

If you were raised female, you might have heard messages focusing on your appearance and not acting up: "You look pretty." "Be a good girl." "You're too emotional."

Many kids also grow up confused and conflicted about their physical functions and capabilities as well as their emotional wants and needs. For example, often kids are trained to contradict their body's innate healing capacity by (a) being told they shouldn't cry, especially boys—the main place boys can express strong emotions is in sports; and (b) being told they should sit still most of the day, despite their natural need to move. Maybe you were told that you shouldn't be so expressive with movement *and* emotions. ("Kids should be seen and not heard.") Activites such as gym and recess have been shortened or taken away altogether, preventing kids from releasing energy, engaging in healthy play with others, or learning to self-regulate with movement. Limiting the healthy connection and expression of your body can keep you cut off from it through adulthood.

How many of us were actually taught about our bodies, feelings, and relationships in such a way that prepared us for real-life encounters as adults? Typically we learned from trial and error because two fundamental aspects of being human—noticing and coping with the full range of emotions and having a body (especially a sexual one)—have been absent from US education *or* primarily focused on potential problems. Can you imagine growing up with courses such as "Introduction to Emotions," "Communication in Relationships," and "Body Awareness 101" as core curriculum in the school of life? If kids aren't learning how to have a healthy relationship with their own physical body and emotions—what we often call the *emotional body*—how can they tune in to the physical body and emotional body of a future partner?

It's not surprising that I see so many clients—independent of age, race, and economic status—who don't trust their bodies. If our actual life experiences aren't validated and mirrored by our caregivers and culture, we later question our inner knowing. This leaves many adults still detached from how their physical or emotional body works, how to listen to it, how to soothe it, how to move it, or what it needs and likes. If you aren't able to listen to your body's various pleasures—to luxuriate and savor them—chances are you won't be able to find satisfaction in the many delightful aspects of life. Instead, you may end up with little capacity to appreciate yourself, heal yourself, connect with your joys, and connect closely with others.

THE KIDS AREN'T ALRIGHT

Things are bound to be better now than when I was growing up in the '80s, right? Not so much. That would be wishful thinking. The ways hypermasculine and hyperfeminine behavior remain separate and encouraged are reflections of society's fears, and its attempts to allay those fears by organizing and simplifying the world. But instead, such separation has created a culture where kids "buy in" to the beliefs that feminine traits—such as empathy, nurturance, compassion, and sharing feelings—aren't valued. Girls are told that their worth is in their appearance and giving enjoyment to others, not themselves, while boys are told that being a man means being powerful and in control. For boys, intimacy has to be about sexuality, not emotions. For girls, intimacy isn't theirs for the taking; it's about the wants and needs of others, not themselves.

If you were raised as a girl, were you focused on "getting" and pleasing the guy? If so, how do you think this prevented you from valuing what *you* wanted in an emotional or physical connection? If you were raised as a boy, were you encouraged to dominate, whether it be on the sports field or in hook-up culture? If so, how do you think this prevented you from being tender and vulnerable? Whatever gender you were socialized as, take some deep breaths as you reflect on this, softening any muscular tension in your body. Imagine the ways you can now take ownership of your full range of emotions and needs—from strong and assertive to gentle and kindhearted.

The journalist Peggy Orenstein's books *Girls and Sex* and *Boys and Sex*, written in 2016 and 2019, respectively, were based on interviews with more than 170 girls and boys, plus academics and experts. She found that boys are being taught to disconnect from their feelings and suppress them, which leads many of them to separate their head from their heart. Whereas girls are being taught to disconnect from their bodies, including their needs, desires, and limits.

The author Glennon Doyle shares a similar theme in her 2020 book *Untamed*, describing the difference she's observed between her son and his male friends and her daughter and her female friends.[3] One afternoon, both groups were hanging out together when she checked on them, asking if they were hungry. The boys said yes, not bothering to turn their attention away from the screen, whereas the girls hesitated and looked to each other first before responding that they were not hungry. What an example of how boys look to inner bodily cues for their needs, while girls look to each other to determine what's acceptable to need. All the mixed messages girls receive about what it means to inhabit a body assigned as female get in the way of other forms of pleasure—everything from food and nourishment to liveliness and desire.

Girls and women are told they're supposed to be the self-sacrificing nurturers for *others*, not driven by their own needs or cravings. A woman is discouraged from acknowledging her own yearnings, whether it be a serving of dessert or an erotic charge for another person. They certainly shouldn't be focused on *their* sensuality or pleasure; if they do, they can be "slut-shamed." As a result, women have traditionally done what they've been taught to value, not what they want. Girls need to learn that how their body wants to feel safe, nurtured, and delighted is just as important—if not more important— than giving that nurturance to others. If you're a parent, help your kids understand what their physical and emotional boundaries are, starting with their likes and dislikes and their need for rest, food, and activity. Encourage saying no to other people's requests when they don't agree with them.

It's hard to make peace with your body's boundaries and pleasures if you aren't acquainted with them in the first place. Many girls turn into women who are still pretty unaware of their body, especially their anatomy. In one program for women, which centered on the reproductive body and sexuality, many participants did not know they even had a clitoris; one woman stated she thought it was the name of a planet. Another woman had no idea she had two different holes—one to urinate and another for menstruation and sexual penetration.[4] The comedian Bridget Christie said, "I was brought up by two very strict Irish Roman Catholics. I've never seen my vagina. I don't want to know what it looks like. I haven't. You know how most parents say to their children, 'Don't look at the sun because you'll go blind'? Ours said that to us but about our genitals."[5] Our language reflects this notion: an old word for a person's genitals (typically female ones) is *pudendum*, which is Latin for "parts to be ashamed of." Whereas the Sanskrit word for vulva is *yoni*, meaning "sacred space." May we all start viewing it as such. And I can pretty much guarantee no one will go blind!

Notice if there are activities and interests related to feeling good in your body (beyond solely sexual enjoyment) that you judge or dismiss because they're "bad" in some way. Do you dismiss them because they're too indulgent, selfish, improper, or time-consuming? Now choose one of these to welcome into your life on a weekly basis, free from guilt or shame, seeing it as an essential part of your self-regulation and life-force energy.

VIOLENCE TO THE PEOPLE

If connecting to your body's desire for life's little pleasures feels too hard, it could be because Americans seem more comfortable with threat and being on guard than relaxation and enjoyment. Here's an example: I was listening to my NPR station as usual and was pleasantly surprised to hear their plan to run a weeklong series on sexual health. The segment began with the announcer warning that the material had sexual content that was not appropriate for younger listeners. This is nothing new, but given that it was sandwiched between a story about a school shooting and one about a civil war, where was the warning about kids hearing violence? We shield our kids from something as natural as physical intimacy and pleasure in their body, yet violence is fair game. For kids and adults alike, I do not get the appeal of all those violent video games, movies, and television shows. The researchers Elaine Hatfield and Richard Rapson point out, "Throughout much of human history, passionate love and sexual desire have been viewed as dangerous, a threat to the social, political, and religious order."[6] So if, as adults, we're afraid of feeling good and believe we have to "protect" ourselves against natural human tendencies, it's no surprise that we pass that along to the next generation.

Males have been told—for centuries—their value lies in strength, domination, and aggression. Orenstein said that when she asked boys to describe their ideal guy, it was all about "stoicism, sexual conquest, dominance, and aggression but to also be chill, athletic, and wealthy. They described building up a wall within them to not feel, to not cry, to not live from their heart; they couldn't show emotional vulnerability."[7] She observed that when boys are together, the way they talk about physical intimacy makes it sound like they are at a construction site: they pound, hammer, nail, smash, and bang. "Young men are still subject to incessant messages that sexual conquest—being always down for sex, racking up their 'body count,' regardless of how they or their partner may feel about it—remains the measure of a 'real man,' and a reliable path to social status."[8] Girls become the objects of these sanctioned violent impulses. After all, any time a person is objectified, they are no longer seen as someone with feelings, deserving of empathy.

The #MeToo movement is evidence that the acceptance of violence and sexual objectification has led to sexual energy becoming a weapon rather than a source of expression and connection. If we want to make our way to a post-#MeToo future, parents and teachers need to support a culture that encourages empathy, communication, caretaking, and cooperation for boys and girls alike. These traits provide the foundation for feeling safe in our bodies and for being able to build healthy pleasures for all types of partnerships—gay, straight, or fluid, long term or casual. It's never too late for you to give your body and emotions some empathy for what you're experiencing. These moments of kindness and self-care are what lead us to collective care.

"LOSING" VIRGINITY

When physical intimacy is discussed with kids in the US, it's been the default to tell them how harmful it could be, leaving out the ways it could be life-enhancing. The phrase *losing your virginity* is one example. The psychologist Doug Braun-Harvey suggests, "Let's encourage, not shame people as they move towards something that is an important developmental milestone."[9] The fixation on our "sexual debut," as he calls it, is couched in right/wrong language. No wonder there are so many adolescents stressed-out about getting their "debut" perfect. So much pressure to do it with the "right" person, at the "right" time and place, and in the "right" way. Braun-Harvey argues that sexual health "is more than just avoiding a negative outcome, sexual health is a *destination* . . . all sexual health definitions are about the balance between pleasure and safety." This potential for growth and connection through intimate relationships is left out of most kids' education.

For my client Judy's mom, there was no such thing as a right person, time, or place, unless it was after marriage. One night when Judy was a junior in high school, she had sex with her boyfriend for the first time. She came home late and was confronted and interrogated by her mom. Judy told the truth about what had happened, and her mom yelled at her and then called her boyfriend's parents. Judy was mortified as she overheard her boyfriend's dad apologize on behalf of his son. This was literally the first time she ever touched on the topic with her mom. Had her mom not been so reactive and punitive, she might have learned that her seventeen-year-old daughter was in a respectful, caring relationship with her boyfriend of several months and that their decision was consensual. (It's worth noting that giving consent does not necessarily mean those involved had a pleasurable time! Sometimes a person gives consent but still feels stress about aspects of the experience.) Rather than *losing* something, we need to reframe someone's first pleasurable sexual experiences as a natural developmental milestone and opportunity for growth.

Most people lacked encouragement on how to derive joy and pleasure from their body in ways that are *not* sexual either. US culture has tended to associate anything related to "touch" as sexual, making it confusing to feel a visceral sensation of joy without wondering if it's inappropriate or slutty. If you're a parent, think of the ways you can encourage your child to embrace their body's pleasurable sensations from appropriate touch, whether it be a hug, hand-holding, or a slow dance.

INACCURATE SEX ED

My Midwest inner-city high school was one of the first in the country to have a clinic that dispensed birth control as well as a daycare center so that young parents could still get their high school diplomas. While in high school, I went to a party at a friend's house. This friend was from a wealthy suburb and was going to a different school. When some of the boys heard about my school's accommodations, they teased me for going to a school where "clearly having the clinic is what led to the need for a daycare." Their ignorance pissed me off. In reality, research shows that abstinence-only programs are connected with higher teen pregnancy rates and don't reduce sexual activity among kids.

Today most states still require sexual education that is abstinence based. Even states that are considered more progressive are focused primarily on risk and danger, avoiding pregnancy, and preventing disease. These 2019 stats from the Guttmacher Institute have found:

- 19 states require emphasis on abstinence before marriage.
- Only 17 states require content to be medically accurate. (*What?!*)
- Only 19 states require information about contraception.
- Only 9 states require culturally appropriate and unbiased information (meaning, not racist, homophobic, or instilling the fear of God).
- Only 3 states restrict the promotion of religion.[10]

Even consent is only taught in eight states (plus Washington, DC) and usually in terms of yet another sexual precaution. According to Orenstein, consent is "another way to dodge more nuanced discussions of personal responsibility, open communication, establishing relationships, understanding gender dynamics and—the third rail of sex ed classes—reciprocal pleasure and the L.G.B.T.Q.+ perspective."[11] Those kinds of conversations are far more nuanced and thoughtful compared to my ninth-grade health class. It was taught by the head football coach, a white man in his fifties, who made us practice putting condoms on bananas and saying the word *penis* out loud with gusto.

MEDIA AS EDUCATOR

In the absence of healthy conversations in the school, do kids learn body positivity and pleasure from their parents? According to a 2017 national survey of three thousand high school students and young adults, "a majority of boys never had a single conversation with their parents about, for instance, how to be sure that your partner wants to be—and is comfortable—having sex with you," or about what it meant to be a respectful sexual partner. About two-thirds had never heard from their parents that they shouldn't have sex with someone who is too intoxicated to consent.[12] The truth is, a child's sexual education defaults to the media.

I've long thought about the role of the media on our well-being. I worked in television news for a couple years after college ("I'm Rachel Allyn with Newscenter 4"), and I wrote a doctoral dissertation about the sexual objectification of women in magazine advertisements. I'll save you the time of reading it and divulge that my results showed women's objectification was getting worse over time, not better. I also found that women of color were more often shown as savage, wearing animal prints, and acting more untamed. Whatever the form of media, it has become both the message and the messenger, able to form children's brains, emotions, and relationships. Kids are curious and will get answers about their growing, changing bodies wherever they can. So naturally they turn to their *smart*phones with easy access to things such as pornography, advertising, and lewd music lyrics despite parents doing their best to manage content.

Due to the prevalence of hard-core pornography, boys and girls are being raised with distorted views of human sexuality. Pornography typically features men dominating women, leading boys to think that's their job in a sexual encounter. If music, television shows, and especially pornography are normalizing brutality and sexual fantasies *for* men, how are boys supposed to develop healthy relationships with women in a culture full of violent, sexually offensive, or demeaning images of women? If advertising uses women's bodies to sell products, then it's not surprising that boys grow up entitled in their domination to "hit on" that or "get a piece of that." Where is the encouragement for males and females to have relationships, including platonic friendships, that are kind, considerate, and playful?

Conversations around the body, intimacy, and sex need to be just as much about discovery, curiosity, and life's pleasures as they are about sexually transmitted infections, pregnancy, and consent. Pleasure is the top reason people of all genders and sexual preferences engage in sexual activity, yet it remains one of the most understudied and undertaught areas of sexual health.

THE THIEF OF JOY

I often think of my fourteen-year-old nephew's experience growing up compared to my own, and how relieved I am that social media wasn't around "back then." I can't imagine being a teenager in an era where everything is recorded and shared for the world to see and critique—braces, acne, and all. Research indicates that increased screen time correlates with anxiety and depression.[13] Who wouldn't feel self-conscious or be riddled with some anxiety after spending hours a day in self-comparison? *Comparison is the thief of joy* after all.

Kids spend so much time online trying to keep up with others that the lines between the real world and the virtual world become blurred. It's like the philosophy question "If a tree falls in the woods and no one hears it, did it really happen?" Except here it's "If it isn't recorded, filtered, uploaded, and liked, did it really happen? And are you really likable, literally?" Life becomes one big act, hiding all the blemishes so common to teenage life. There is the saying, "You can't be what you can't see," and if kids don't see real life, they'll think there's something wrong with them. Let's see more expressions of joy and pleasure in various forms like the silly mishaps, the adventures, and the awkwardness.

The very nature of social media is that it preys on people's insecurity, triggering envy and FOMO (fear of missing out). It's practically the very definition of fake news by creating "falsehoods"—false identities in which your appearance and activities are edited and inauthentic. No amount of social media followers can remedy this feeling of not being good enough, pretty enough, interesting enough, simply as you are. This is like kryptonite to cultivating body love on the path to developing a bodyful life. Maybe there should be warnings on some of these apps like there are on cigarettes?

Whether it be social media or porn, kids are socially isolated as they watch, cut off from relating to others. I worry about all the missed opportunities to practice making real connections with real people. If social media becomes children's primary way of connecting with the world, how will they learn important subtle interpersonal cues and compassionate listening between peers? These are building blocks for pleasurable connection between three-dimensional humans.

NATURE DEFICIT DISORDER

Nielsen ratings note that in the US, children and adults spend an average of six hours a day sitting still in front of some kind of screen or monitor. "The average American child is said to spend four to seven minutes a day in unstructured play outdoors, and more than seven hours a day in front of a screen."[14] This crisis has led to what is known as *nature deficit disorder*. Being outside is so necessary and beneficial, for kids and adults. It can promote confidence, creativity, and stimulation. It gets the body moving and helps reduce stress. The solution? Get moving, ideally outside. I always say, *movement is medicine.* Engaging in a diverse variety of movement activities is what our bodies yearn for. Kids and adults alike benefit from:

- Team sports to connect and support each other with shared goals.
- Daily yoga, stretching, and other types of moving meditations.
- Keeping gym and recess in schools everyday.
- Getting outside as much as possible, ideally every day.
- Biking versus driving to work, school, or errands.

From the beginning of time we've been creatures who danced and sang. Then we got increasingly "buttoned up." I suggest you dance and shake out the old body memory full of constricting messages and release your unique voice to connect with your true self. Pick your favorite song(s) that inspires movement and let yourself be carefree in your body.

COME "OUT" OF WHAT?

In junior high, my girlfriends and I would suffer through moments in the hallway when a boy would sneak up behind us and snap our bras or "pants" us (yanking down our skirt or shorts). Back then it was considered "boys being boys," whereas today most schools would consider this as a very serious offense. I also hear friends with teenagers talk about their kids' increased acceptance for gender fluidity, whether it be someone's sexuality, being transgender, or a preferred pronoun (she/her, he/him, or they/them). One of my friends asked her seventh-grade daughter if she knew any kids at school who had "come out" as gay. Her daughter didn't understand the question, replying, "What is there to come out of? If boys like boys and girls like girls, it's no big deal."

The way we categorize boys and girls, and the way culture lumps all forms of pleasure into sexual conquest, thwarts all the other ways we can embrace life's pleasures—such as those found in the senses and in nature, creativity and play, or in moments of liveliness and flow states—and makes bodyfulness all the more challenging. I worry that kids sometimes miss out on the sweet, tender pleasures found in a slow dance, the first hand-holding, or snuggling under the stars.

Freeing ourselves from limited ideas of who we're supposed to be involves a retraining of sorts. Alongside the bodyful practices I'll talk about, we need to help kids develop emotional intelligence. Educating them on the ways emotions can show up in their body, and how to acknowledge and share those emotions, is an invaluable skill—and one that's never too late to start learning. There is a lot of power in simply helping kids acknowledge how they're feeling with kindness, which I explain more in the next chapter with the practice of "tending and befriending." Invite conversations with your children about connecting to their emotions, curiosities, and the wide array of pleasures outside of the bedroom that can inspire moments of bliss and human connection.

UNCHANGING ESSENCE

Buried beneath the conflicting messages about the body, our gender, and our relationships remains a primal, natural part of ourselves. I call this our *unchanging essence*. It has nothing to do with external things—such as how much money we have, how much we weigh, how many social media followers we have, or whether we're partnered or single—which can change in an instant due to anything from a recession to a bout of stomach flu. When I think of my own unchanging essence, I think of the special place in my heart for animals, my love of international travel, my joy in being barefoot, and my thirst for karaoke. As you reflect on your unchanging essence, think back to anytime you've felt more at ease, even going back to childhood.

Hopefully you can rediscover parts of yourself that may have been buried. As the writer and entrepreneur Emily McDowell puts it, "Finding yourself is not really how it works. You aren't a ten-dollar bill in last winter's coat pocket. You are also not lost. Your true self is right there, buried under cultural conditioning, other people's opinions, and inaccurate conclusions you drew as a kid that became your beliefs about who you are. Finding yourself is actually returning to yourself. An unlearning, an excavation, a remembering who you were before the world got its hands on you." The weight of repression, violence, superficiality, and disconnection can become a heavy load to carry. But it's never too late to unpack that weight.

I'm not the "kind of woman" who is supposed to talk about things such as pleasure, sex, body fluids, or desire. I'm certainly not supposed to be speaking about it on stage or writing a book about it. This is not what "good girls" do. In which case I'm proud to be my bad self. You could say I have a habit of being utterly *me*. Being bodyful and having a life of healthy pleasures requires breaking free from categories telling us who we *should* be rather than who we truly are. And who we truly are is human in all the ways we are meant to express it, not robots easily defined, confined, categorized, and objectified. We may not always understand the experience of bodies different from us—male-bodied people don't know the experience of fear that lives in female-bodied people, just as heterosexual bodies don't know the experience of judgement of nonheterosexual bodies—but we can start with respecting all bodies, in all ways, seeing beauty in the difference.

Getting woke to pleasure starts by stepping into your own unique essence within you, the very thing you were taught as a child to control, suppress, and assign goofy anatomical names for. It starts by reclaiming your body and noticing all it does for you. This reclamation isn't just about the outer look—although it's fantastic to like your appearance, of course—it's about appreciating the miraculous ecosystem of your body. It's about treating it with care every single day. Because this body with its pulsing heart is the ultimate portal to the inner wisdom, acceptance, and expression we all want yet feel estranged from.

~ 5 ~

Not Tonight, Honey,
I'd Rather Instagram

It takes courage to say yes to rest and play in a
culture where exhaustion is seen as a status symbol.
—*Brené Brown*

I'VE CERTAINLY HAD my moments of being a stress case, detached
from my body, unable to experience life's pleasures—or even notice
when they present themselves. In my last year of graduate school,
I was working full time at an inner-city hospital considered a "level
one" trauma center while trying to finish my dissertation, apply for
post-doctoral positions, and maintain a long-distance relationship.
I could put myself into high gear by day, but I couldn't turn off at
night. I had heard about Ambien and it became my wonder drug—
goodbye neurotic nighttime musings, hello rest! Until . . .

One morning I woke up feeling oddly full. I walked into the
kitchen to find it in disarray with wrappers and crumbs strewn every-
where. Had a squirrel invaded? And then I began to faintly remember something about salad croutons and pretzels (apparently the only
carbohydrates in the house). This happened a few more times, each
episode leaving me disturbed that I didn't remember my behavior. It
even happened when I visited my partner; he would see the evidence
in his kitchen and tell me, "You've gone cuckoo for Cocoa Puffs again."

Since that time, fifteen years ago, it's become common knowledge that if you don't go straight to bed after taking Ambien you run
the risk of doing all sorts of things unconsciously, such as driving,
sending emails, raiding the refrigerator, or even having sex. My brief

Ambien adventures confirmed my belief that when you tamper with one bodily system, you're messing with another. A major side effect of antidepressants, for example, is sexual dysfunction (which could exacerbate the depression). Seems counterproductive! The public policy professor Paul Batalden once said, "Every system is perfectly designed to get the results it gets."[1] This includes the body. Yet we mess with it all the time.

Our overmedicalized culture tries to override our natural state. Like I had done with Ambien, people avoid or hide from their challenging feelings with pills, bypassing more time-consuming strategies that help them learn to cope with hard feelings and situations. In my case, the meds were a flimsy bandage over the deeper wound of why I felt too stressed to sleep. These ways of tampering with our bodies and ignoring the underlying imbalances can have lasting effects. In my case, I gained weight from my nighttime food fests, became reliant on a pill full of chemicals, and delayed getting to the heart of my sleeplessness.

More than ever, people are choosing distractions instead of finding ways to deal with life's problems head-on by processing and releasing emotions and making lifestyle changes. Just look at the opioid epidemic. And although plant medicine substances, such as marijuana, are more natural than pharmaceuticals, people can also become overly reliant on them to numb out. The legalization of pot has made it easier to get the high to help you sleep, relax, or giggle. Recently in California, where it's legal, I had a moment while sitting at a cafe sipping my matcha when I looked around and suddenly a light bulb went off; everyone was high except me. I couldn't prove this, but my Spidey sense is pretty accurate. By being sober, I was the odd one out. Whether it be Ambien or marijuana, they're both ways to *escape* the realities of your mind and body, which certainly doesn't foster genuine intimacy. What are we trying so hard to get away from?

STRESS BY THE NUMBERS

Statistics tell a rather grim tale of Americans working and worrying more, playing and relaxing less. Applauding busyness and disparaging rest. Turning on their screens and tuning out each other. Plugging into what's going on around the world 24/7 and yet, ironically, feeling lonelier than ever. Facing barriers and inequities in getting treatment for our mental and physical health and suffering as a result. We're a nation of people disconnected from our bodies, dissatisfied in our relationships, frustrated at work, and unable to slow down enough to enjoy our lives a bit more.

In a culture that values productivity over pleasure, profits over people, and the superficial over the authentic, there are physical, emotional, and financial consequences. We place unrealistic expectations on ourselves and others—"If I just work hard enough I could have it all"—at the expense of balance, vitality, and intimacy. Lovers are literally turning on their phones instead of their partners at bedtime. People struggle with high levels of self-criticism, poor body image, and addictions to medications, all of which rob them from experiencing mental and physical ease and life's natural pleasures. There are also public health implications. Let's look at the stats.

LESS VACATION TIME

We may think we're working harder and producing more by taking fewer vacations but, in fact, numerous studies show that less vacation time results in lower work productivity. Workers in France average twenty-five to thirty days of paid vacation time, which is fifteen to twenty days more than workers in the US, and productivity in France is higher.[2] A 2017 Gallup poll showed that Americans take 70 percent fewer vacations since 2001, and even if they do take time away from work for a national holiday, half of them check in with the office, which gets in the way of their ability to decompress and refresh.[3] Perhaps people feel the need to work so much in the US because their health care and retirement are linked to their jobs rather than being fundamental rights as citizens. For some workaholics, it took getting furloughed during the COVID-19 pandemic to finally take a moment for rest and relaxation. One of the reasons I lead weeklong retreats is because it typically takes much more than just a weekend for people to unwind enough to feel restored. There's nothing *wrong* with being productive and loving your job, of course; that can be a pleasure all its own, especially if you derive meaning from your work and get into flow states, but not when it comes at the expense of rest, relationships, and sanity.

This is a friendly reminder to take *all* your allotted vacation time. Done right (truly not working!), you'll calm your nervous system and reconnect with pleasurable aspects of your personal life.

FEWER CONNECTIONS

This digital era has become the disconnected era, separating us from our bodies and each other. We've become like my Bluetooth when it's unable to sync with my speaker: "Paired but not connected." Humans are wired for connection, yet many Americans are lonelier than ever, which research shows can be deadly. Forced isolation, like we experienced during COVID-19, can be a contributing factor to what's known as "deaths of despair"—death by drugs, alcohol, and suicide that result from the combination of economic uncertainty and loneliness.[4] This could become a type of pandemic all its own. One comprehensive study found that the impact of social isolation, living alone, and loneliness can lead to risk of early mortality, on par with factors such as obesity and smoking.[5] Our separateness is not only distressing but also costly. Public health statistics show that mental health issues, such as anxiety and depression, are the most expensive medical conditions in the country and serious mental illness costs Americans $193.2 billion in lost earnings per year.[6]

Real connection goes beyond having followers on social media, getting little dopamine hits from all the "likes" and comments. It means letting ourselves be known in *real* life and wanting to know others more deeply. If we're looking at screens instead of each other, not making eye contact, we aren't cultivating "mirror neurons," the brain chemicals that promote empathy and compassion, which we need more than ever. Beyond survival, the connection that comes from genuine relationships is tied to confidence, meaning, and purpose, all aspects of feeling like we matter; which is key to loving our body and owning our right to healthy pleasures.

When overworking and technology cause us to become disconnected from ourselves, we lose the ability to be in touch with how we feel or how to modulate the feelings we do notice. It means we're not in touch with what our bodies need to be healthy. This can lead to secondary problems such as addictive behaviors, critical thoughts, acting impulsively, and other ways of mistreating ourselves. And, of course, not knowing how to take care of ourselves impacts our ability to be in healthy relationships with others.

Practice the "Body Conversation" exercise at the end of the book. It can help you develop awareness about your body language to stay informed of your emotions and corresponding feelings and to stay balanced.

LESS SEX

Who has the time or the desire for any kind of intimacy when work is piling up, screen time trumps one-on-one time, and nothing is more appealing at the end of the day than the chance to get a good night's sleep? Turns out, fewer of us these days. According to a 2017 study in the *Archives of Sexual Behavior*, American adults had sex approximately nine fewer times a year in the early 2010s than they did in the late 1990s.[7] The results showed this to be true across most demographic variables—race, gender, religion, work status, and education level. Oddly enough, Generation Z and the millennials had less sex than those over age seventy, who were busy keeping the flame lit. The drop was even more stark among married couples—who got it on only fifty-five times (approximately) in 2014 compared to seventy-three times in 1990.[8] Researchers attributed the drop in desire to longer work hours, increased use of pornography, helicopter parenting, increased chronic pain, side effects from medication, and overuse of screen time. The notable sex therapist Pepper Schwartz argues that the number one reason for people's declining sex lives is fatigue.[9]

Speaking of porn, research shows that those who watch it regularly feel less satisfaction in their own partnered relationships. People are more critical of their body, their partner's body, and their sexual performance overall; it distorts what sexual acts people *think* they should engage in because it emphasizes showmanship and performance.[10] Where are the media messages of vulnerability, tenderness, mutuality, and respect so essential to healthy intimate relationships? Instead we glamorize sex as getting off, showing off, and boosting our ego.

In the immortal words of Tina Turner, "What's Love Got to Do with It?" Apparently not much, in a culture that loves money even more. The author Kristen Ghodsee researched what happened to women in countries that transitioned from socialism to capitalism and found that women reported better sex under socialism.[11] Ghodsee argues that capitalism harms women more than men with its narrative to "have it all." The reality is that working full time at the office, trying to break the glass ceiling—while dealing with a wage gap, harassment, and discrimination—and then doing the bulk of the housework and childcare doesn't exactly boost the libido.

These statistics are an important reminder that *nothing is wrong with you* for being too exhausted by all your demands to engage intimately at times. So often clients have shared with me their guilt for not being in "in the mood" or, conversely, feeling rejected by a partner who wasn't. Whichever camp you fall in, I'll share my ideas for handling mismatched desires in part three.

MORE SCREEN TIME

Here's a mind-boggling statistic: there's an estimated 2.5 billion (with a *b*!) smartphones currently in use.[12] Cell phones alone distract people an average of eighty times per day in the US.[13] With numbers like that, it's no surprise that the digital world is overtaking our connection to the human world. Although there are benefits to having the information superhighway at our fingertips, there are clearly drawbacks. Social media seduces us. It certainly becomes easier to stay at home, plug in, and not connect with others in real life. When we do venture out, we tend to make less eye contact and be less inclined to notice what's going on around us. In the competition for our attention, we're often not paying attention to much of anything, carelessly missing out on our surroundings.

Our mass migration to the indoors, and to the screens inside our four walls, has left us zoned out with hunched-over "tech necks," furrowed brows, and achy bodies yearning to move, stretch, and engage. I mentioned in the last chapter that nature deficit disorder is becoming a real issue for kids; well, it's an issue for adults too. Nature deficit disorder is associated with depression, loss of empathy, and lack of altruism,[14] whereas time in nature is associated with a positive mood, psychological well-being, meaningfulness, and vitality.[15] But nature can only help us feel bodyful if we're actually *in* the natural world and not distracted playing music, listening to podcasts, or talking on our cell phones. Let's find ways to bust through this "fourth wall" of our screens inside our homes and get our butts outside.

How has technology affected your attention (and intentions) throughout the day? Think about how you can stay present to the "offline" moments of your life, such as having an undistracted conversation or silently enjoying an outside view.

I've learned that if you have your own business, social media can be an effective way to promote your brand (and it seems everyone is their own brand these days). But it's a double-edged sword; we now know how Big Media is an attention vampire, polarizing us and selling our data. Ironically, it wasn't lost on me that I was spending a massive amount of time sitting in front of a computer to write this book and attempting to keep up my business on social media while critiquing overuse of screen time. My body was breaking down from all that sitting and computer-staring, giving literal meaning to me being a "wounded healer." Moderation with screens comes naturally as long as I'm engaging in the real world with the people I care about. Unless it's TikTok. I'll confess there's something delightfully addictive about those snippets of dancing and lip-syncing, a nice counterbalance to the negative news out there.

IT'S ME TIME

Moderation is a skill to cultivate in many aspects of our modern era, including moderating pleasure. The alternatives—restricting or bingeing on things—can cause more problems. The main area where I see people trying to reclaim balance (with rest, enjoyment, self-validation)—and not always succeeding—is with food, one of our earliest relationships. Picture this: My client Paula will try to be "good" all day, whether it be with her eating, workouts, productivity at the office, or supporting her friends, coworkers, and family. Paula essentially spends the day giving, giving, giving, and restraining, restraining, restraining. Then the kids go to sleep and she devours a big bag of cookies with too much wine and feels bad about herself.

My interpretation is that Paula has the "naughty" food or drink as her way of saying "It's finally me time!" We can only exert so much willpower all day, day after day, over so many things. By evening, when we're tired, our inner voice that says "What the hell, I deserve to receive too" gets louder. So we do something indulgent as a way of saying, "You're right. I matter too." When Paula sprinkles in some nurturing escapes throughout her week and relaxes her unrealistic expectations for herself in all areas of her life, she's less likely to have an explosion of gluttony later on that she feels guilty about. We also explored where the beliefs came from that she has to be Mother Teresa to everyone except herself in order to be a "good" person.

"NEVER ENOUGH" SYNDROME

On the flip side of being overly restrained is too much consumption. For starters, we are all media consumers, almost constantly bombarded with messages that tell us how we should look and act, and with invitations to buy products that purport to help us achieve that.

So we seek validation from outside of ourselves, trying to find it in "stuff." We think the nice car and bigger house will give us happiness and status. There's always an upgrade around the corner that we think we can't live without.

I happen to have an Apple watch. I can't tell you how many times I'll look down at my wrist to check the time and instead it's stuck on a screen of recent texts, my last-played podcast, or anything but the time. I find myself pressing buttons, eventually getting so frustrated I exclaim, "Why can't you just be a watch?!" Some things we think will bring us more convenience—which we want because we're so darn busy—create just the opposite. Consumer culture stands in opposition to rejoicing in simple everyday pleasures that already exist with us and around us. The best things in life aren't things.

Recall an experience, rather than a material object, that elicits fond memories. What did this entail on a sensory level? Did you share it with someone else? What do you cherish about that experience?

The expectations we put on ourselves to "have it all," whether that means material possessions or status, are impossible to achieve. It's an endless maze that rarely brings the joy we anticipate. Instead it leads to what I call the "never enough" syndrome. We think we'll be happy when we lose those ten pounds, get that promotion at work, or have more followers on social media, but these things outside of us are fleeting and, even if they are attainable, they're never quite enough. What is lasting, affordable, and accessible is your breath, your body's capacity to heal through self-soothing behaviors, and your intentions. I'll talk more about this in part two.

NEW SHOES AND NEW BOOS

Americans place wealth, status, and clout above everything, with beauty, fashion, and youth a close second. As a culture of seekers, always looking to optimize ourselves, another way we consume is through self-improvement (and we've all seen examples of self-improvement gone wrong). Since physical attraction is associated with youth, we try to defy aging with skin creams, diets, and over-the-top products.

Here's an absurd example of body commodification in the name of modern "beauty." While I was with a friend at the hilariously named The Smitten Kitten, an adult toy shop, we noticed they were selling adhesive nipples for women who wanted to turn their "headlights" on. They even had a sample out, so naturally I couldn't resist putting it on between my T-shirt and sweater. I certainly looked perky on that side. We got a good chuckle out of it, then continued to shop, parted ways, and I resumed some errands.

That night I got home, took off my sweater, and the sample nipple fell out! Not only did I accidentally steal it but I'd gone all over town with it on, "smuggling raisins" as we used to say, except in this case smuggling a raisin. I drove back to the store to return it and apologize, but when I pulled up, I suddenly couldn't find the sample. I ransacked my car. It must have fallen out somewhere between my house and car. If this little fake nipple is ever found, someone will be in for a surprise.

This is just a little example (literally) of the beauty extremes people resort to. Whether it be nipple enhancers, eyelash extensions, acrylic nails, hair dyes, tanning booths, lip plumping, or Botox, our beauty standards keep people in a hamster wheel of never-ending self-improvement. The self-improvement industry counts on us constantly "buying new shoes and looking for new boos." Where did the modern, mainstream definition of beauty even come from? White men in positions of power and white culture overall, which certainly doesn't represent all bodies and races in the US. And it's an industry that keeps people caught in self-loathing, distracted from their inner beauty and strength. If this feels familiar to you, maybe it's time you stop being a bully to yourself and reclaim your inner bombshell. Recognize and appreciate how your body shows up for you like a boss every day and bow down to her majesty.

Ask yourself how you "buy in" to these cultural myths that tell you looking like "an influencer" gives you more worth? And how does that distract you from recognizing the infinite potential in your body at this moment?

We've become superficial, judging people on their pedigree or appearance, not on their heart and soul. What if people became influencers on social media not because they could gyrate in a midriff top but because they were compassionate, insightful, and generous . . . because they used their brilliance to help others shine? If these were the traits we truly valued in our culture, humanitarians would be as wealthy and recognizable as celebrities.

Constant self-criticism is exhausting and distracts you from your potential. Counter that lack with some love. For every criticism you tell yourself ("my stomach is flabby"), follow it up with the opposite ("my love handles are sexy").

SEX SELLS

Cultural messages ping-pong between treating the body's pleasures as taboo (our puritanical roots) and exploiting the body to sell products (our capitalist culture). "Sex sells," as the advertising world is fond of telling us (as though it were a good thing), which really means that the industry commodifies people's bodies in salacious ways to sell an image (young, beautiful, fit, free, sexy). After decades of women being sexually objectified, I've noticed that some are taking back control of their own image. While a younger woman might do that because she thinks it's the only way she'll get attention, an older, more seasoned woman might find it empowering. It's tricky.

Sex sells because we yearn for the passions of the taboo. And if we're too busy or ashamed to tend to our natural needs within the every day, and with three-dimensional people, then pent-up impulses get satisfied with screens and shopping instead. What you're really buying is a hedonistic hit of instant gratification, an illusion of something lasting. Yet genuine conversations about emotional and physical intimacy are not shown as much in the media; apparently the sweeter or more sobering aspects of life don't get high ratings.

Judging from the rather dismal picture these stories and statistics paint, we've become a culture of overachieving consumers stuck in our heads. Modern-day barriers prevent us from being connected to our bodies, our real selves, and one another. The fact is we want to reconnect, we want more fulfilling relationships, and we want to feel pleasure in our bodies free from shame and embarrassment—in real time, in real life. But we don't quite know how. So how do we find whole-person health in an unhealthy world? How do we become connected—to our own radiance and to the light in others—within a deeply divisive culture? It starts with remembering that you are not broken; the societal systems are.

TEND AND BEFRIEND

Start by seeing how hard it is to be a human these days. There is so much power in self-acknowledgment when it's gentle and warm-hearted. Begin by connecting to your emotions, the visceral messengers that inform what you identify as feelings.

Many people don't realize that emotions and feelings are interconnected but they're not the same. Feelings are sparked by emotions. For example, you might notice the emotion of discomfort while at a party as your stomach clenches and your breathing gets constricted. Then your mind labels that emotion as "awkward" because [*insert story line: perhaps you don't know many people or you saw an ex . . . and away your mind goes*]. One person's awkward could be another person's excitement about meeting new people. This is why feelings can be so different from person to person in the same scenario. Take a different example of emotional threat: a bully might respond with the feeling of anger, because it feels empowering and labeling it "fear" would be too vulnerable. In contrast, the non-bully would respond with a feeling of anxiety. Your emotions tell it like it is; your mental feelings are the ones who can get gossipy and create binaries (this is good/bad, right/wrong). Listening to your bodily emotions, informed by your sense perception as I'll discuss more in chapter 10, helps you connect to the reality of your present experience.

Everything we experience is part of a larger cycle. Day and night, sun and moon, rest and activity, and, of course, life and death. But most people forget about the emotional cycle because they never learned to appreciate the wisdom emotions offer and how to integrate them in their life. This blocks us from a wise language within, which is always trying to give us useful information to stay regulated.

The body nailed emotional expression long before Shakespeare—tears, laughter, jealousy, heartache—an actor playing their part on the stage of your body. Because humans naturally avoid pain, it's normal to chase the pleasant emotions and avoid the prickly ones. What we end up doing is avoiding these brilliant messengers and seeking the quickest refuge possible outside of ourselves, which creates a new layer of problems (overspending, overeating, overcriticizing . . .). So the hurdle becomes the overreliance on these distractions to *not* feel. Our emotions are for emoting, our feelings are for feeling—not for repressing or denying. From an evolutionary perspective, it's the full range of emotions that have protected and guided humans by leading to awareness and thoughtful decision-making.

We also hide our feelings from others. We live in an emotionally private culture for fear of offending someone or being judged. How often have you gone through the motions when someone says, "How are you?" by responding "I'm fine" even when the truth is that you're *not* fine at all! Unless you define it as I once heard: code for **F**ucked-up, **I**nsecure, **N**eurotic, and **E**motional. If someone was that honest with you, your jaw would probably drop (sure, it might be a lot to throw at someone while in passing at the market). I wish people felt more comfortable "keeping it real." We not only hold back sharing our emotions, we also avoid talking about topics that *elicit* emotions, such as death, sex, money, and race, despite being important aspects of life and topics that could create deeper understanding.

Connecting to your raw emotions is a profound way to "tend and befriend" yourself, also referred to with yet another catchy rhyme, "to name it is to tame it." How it works: pause, take expansive breaths, and notice where the emotions are in your body. If you're confused by how emotions manifest inside of you, refer to the "Language of Sensations Handout" at the end of the book for examples. Then bring your hand to that area (perhaps the heart or abdomen) and release any muscular constriction. Breathing can help with that release. Ask what your emotions are trying to tell you? Do they have something valuable to share? In what way could this emotion be a useful signal to you? Then name the feeling(s) you associate with your bodily emotions. Don't try to change or fix them, just observe and name them. Breathe in and out this acknowledgment as both an act of kindness and, as I'll share more in chapter 7, a way to regulate your nervous system. Now notice if you would feel better by shaking, stretching, or sighing out the energy of that emotion, or if staying still and softening into the emotions and corresponding feelings is more helpful. Explore this subtle but powerful practice every day.

One of my clients talked about becoming a junior professional swimmer by age 14, an alcoholic by age 18, a recovering addict by age 22, a mom at 24, and a graduate student at 28. Here she was, trying to figure out for the first time *who* she was aside from the labels of athlete, addict, mom, and law student. "Who am I, what do I want, and what do I feel?" were foreign concepts to her. We focused on her slowing down, getting out of her overthinking mind, and drawing her attention to the emotions in her body. From there she practiced tending and befriending them so she could identify, appreciate, and live from her own truth and not old limiting labels.

This exercise can help alleviate the discord people feel between who they are and who they think they should be. It drops the insidious voice of comparison. After all, if you're not living from your essence, who are you being? Sadly, many people are trying to be *other* people.

JOMO

In a society that sees time as one of our most valuable currencies, we're always seeking shortcuts. So it goes with our communication—verbal or digital. I find the acronyms in the online dating world the most humorous: preferences such as NOS (no one-night stands) or FWB (friends with benefits); descriptors such as HWP (height-weight proportionate) and MBA (married but available). At least they're being honest—on the app, that is; their partner, on the other hand, may be in the dark. There are also shortcuts to specify which reality we're referring to (IRL is in real life) and feelings, such as FOMO (fear of missing out).

It's been said that life is what happens when you're busy making other plans—and also while you're zoned out in front of a screen. Every second of every day there are people doing hilarious, raunchy, and ridiculous things for you to marvel at online. It can leave you feeling that your life isn't nearly as cool. But all that glitters isn't gold; the filters and editing on social media can turn anyone's experience from trashy to classy. As an overzealous person often prone to FOMO, I had to embrace the saying "You can do anything but you can't do everything."

You can only do so much at once. The frenzy to produce and achieve all the time can work against you. Sometimes I have to stop and remind myself to cool my jets because I'm not late, I'm just accustomed to *thinking* I am. The irony is I have become increasingly late to things despite rushing around. I cram in that extra text or laundry folding because it gives me the illusion that I'm winning the race against the clock. But what I'm really sacrificing is peace of mind and body; and the more I hurry, the more I drop or misplace things anyway. Haste makes waste.

Join me in adopting the alternate to FOMO, JOMO (joy of missing out)—especially if you are beleaguered by expecting yourself to "do it all." Being able to let go and appreciate where you're at, amid all the options, provides a peaceful pleasure all its own. You could call this JOPO (joy of pleasuring out). Okay, enough of the acronyms.

Practice noticing how good it can feel to say no in order to say yes to what you really need in the moment.

EPICUREAN LIFESTYLE

If American culture valued rest, healthy relationships and pleasures, and all bodily shapes, sizes, and skin colors, we wouldn't have to swim upstream to feel whole. Perhaps we could live a more *epicurean* lifestyle. The word has come to mean the pursuit of pleasure with food, comforts, and other luxuries, but epicurean philosophy is really about encouraging simple pleasures as a way to find tranquility.

Named after the Greek Epicurus, and dating back to 307 B.C.E., the epicurean lifestyle encourages minimalist living and rejoicing in the natural world. Early epicureans saw all the striving and angst to consume more, more, more as pointless. Which reminds me of another Greek, Sisyphus, who, according to the mythological story, was constantly pushing a boulder up a mountain only to have it fall back down to the bottom every time he'd approach the top. Hardships are the hallmark of a very different philosophy, Stoicism, which encourages the endurance of pain or adversity without showing emotions or complaining.

Early epicureans felt nature designed humans to seek and receive pleasures, but not to excess. To help people discern among all the pleasurable options, Epicurus divided them into three categories: (1) natural and necessary—eating, drinking, sleeping, shelter, and social interactions; (2) natural and not necessary—sex, having children, and being held in high esteem by others; and (3) not natural and not necessary—good ol' vices and things that are "bad" for you, such as vanity, greed, and drugs.

Ask yourself: "Was I raised in an environment that was more stoic, epicurean, or a balance of the two? Was I given messages that pleasure was an indulgence or an unproductive waste of time? Were there manipulative strings attached if I gave myself pleasure, play, rest? Did my household model a balance of work and play, of self-discipline and relaxation?"

During the COVID-19 pandemic, I initially found myself "deteriorating faster than I could lower my standards," as the writer Anne Lamott put it. Then I got a grip and used that big moment of pause to savor some simple things like an epicurean. I began to cherish my daily walks, stopping to smell the lilac bushes. The routine of my shower became more luxurious, with scrubs and nice body lotion afterward (and then there were days I couldn't be bothered with much hygiene at all, a rare pleasure I also discovered during this time). In the absence of going to events and restaurants at night, dinner became more sacred, and I delighted in eating a variety of ethnic cuisines. And while meeting a friend over video chat wasn't nearly as sweet as hugging them and sharing space, I felt more gratitude than ever for having them in my life. If we stop trying to be so "extra," with fancy stuff and pursuits, we notice that the wonder of life is in its beautiful ordinariness.

Make a list of five epicurean pleasures you can invite into your weekly routine as pleasure breaks.

My office, classrooms, and retreats provide sacred space for those with stories of disconnection—whether it be with food, community, their body, or their partner. I listen as they describe the search for ease or passion—key aspects of a satisfying life. You don't have to be a therapist to see the harried ways Americans seek quick pleasures in their attempt to avoid discomfort but somehow cause themselves more suffering along the way.

We've become so accustomed to stimulation—our attention is diverted by dings, requests, comparisons, and consumption; our nervous systems are on constant alert. Our overloaded brains and bodies can only handle so much. No wonder people turn to Ambien, marijuana, alcohol, or other sedatives in an attempt to slow down or protest the chaos.

What can we do with this crap we've been dealt? I've been focusing in the last few chapters on the barriers to bodyful pleasure, not to wag my finger at you but to help you see that *you* are not the problem, these barriers don't define you, and you can choose to break them down or refuse to believe they exist. You don't have to "buy in" *or* "lean in." You have agency to exit the rat race. Whole-body health comes from living *well*, which takes intention and courage. Serenity is right there inside you, but first you need to turn off your smartphone and judging mind.

~

PART TWO

The Body
Holds the Key

~ 6 ~

Body. Full. Ness.: Not Your Mother's Mindfulness

There is one thing, that when cultivated and regularly practiced, leads to deep spiritual intention, to peace, to mindfulness and clear comprehension, to vision and knowledge, to a happy life here and now, and to the culmination of wisdom and awakening. And what is that one thing? It's mindfulness centered on the body.

—Buddha

IF I WERE TO offer you a life hack it would be this: *There are no life hacks.* Almost everything meaningful comes with patience and practice. The closest thing I can offer you is this: your body is meant to move, so *move your body.* No one would dispute that exercising has all sorts of health benefits; it prevents obesity, reduces heart disease, and strengthens your muscles and bones. But science is revealing how essential body movement is to our emotional health as well. Feeling angry? Shake it out. Feeling grief? Bawl it out. Feeling happy? Dance it out. Feeling worried? Run it out. Or bike, bounce, twist, groan, swim, bend, roll . . . because your ability to move therapeutically is a medicine you were born with. Your healing is in your hands, literally. This is the panacea we all possess to be able to reside in this body of ours with more pleasure and joy.

YOUR BODY IS NOT BAGGAGE

Accessing this postnatal medicine begins when you commit to trusting your body instead of controlling or ignoring it. It's common for people to drag their body around wherever their mind goes, practically forgetting it's there. That thing you're schlepping is actually an expansive ecosystem to be marveled at. Like Santa's elves at the North Pole, each doing their part to pull off Christmas, all the organisms of your body join together to pull off your daily lived experience.

An ecosystem is defined as "a community of living organisms in conjunction with the nonliving components of their environment, interacting as a system. These biotic and abiotic components are linked together through nutrient cycles and energy flows."[1]

The hallmark of any ecosystem is that positive change in one area often leads to improvements overall. What if you had new tools within you to start a wave of improvement, to keep your emotions and energy regulated, and prevent moments of *dis*-ease in your life from becoming full-blown physical disease? The fact is, you do. *Bodyfulness.*

FOREIGN BODY

Not to be confused with how full you feel after your Thanksgiving meal, *bodyful* means connecting to your whole body *fully*, in a way that leaves you *full*-filled. But all wordplay and one fewer *l* aside, bodyfulness is an innovative way to relate to your body that can reignite sparks of ease and pleasure in your life. I believe its combination of inquiry, engagement, and release can get to the heart of things more deeply than talk therapy, medication, or exercise alone.

How do I explain this? Over time there have been two main issues that I've seen come up repeatedly in my work: First, the extent to which people are disconnected and stressed is huge. My clients know this but struggle with *how* to find ease and connection again. Second, as soon as we fold in breathing and moving we're able to go further with their psychological processing. By inviting the body into the conversation, I've noticed clients become more raw and experience deeper release and repair in *and* out of our sessions. As far as I'm concerned, that's precisely what they're coming to me for.

I've also seen students in my yoga-psychology workshops release tears or built-up agitation during and after class. They tell me later they felt tension unleash followed by a sense of spaciousness, as if something stuck inside their body was set free. Over time and with practice, I see them tolerate that initial discomfort of being in their body when hard emotions arise and then be able to pacify them with recognition, discharge, and kindness. It's visceral moments like these that help people start to discover the potential of a body-up approach to heal their head and heart.

I've watched many intelligent people walk in and out of my office. I've helped facilitate and been witness to their insights, wisdom that they've rediscovered within themselves, only to notice a gap between their revelations and their later actions. What causes this gap between the light bulb in their head and the change in their behavior? It's simple—so simple that we've overlooked it: they were not able to *em-body* the new insights. Their transformation gets stuck in their head where it sits in the "bottleneck" between their head and their heart, between their mind (with constructed versions of reality) and their inner visceral memory. We sure do put a lot of pressure on those minds of ours to do *everything*; to be a one-stop shop for healing ourselves, and perhaps the world! But when there's communication and cooperation throughout the entire ecosystem of the body and mind, things click. This is a different kind of intelligence, one that encourages more lasting change.

My challenge is that many people see their body as something foreign rather than as a friend. Which isn't surprising, given messages throughout US history and the modern distractions I talked about in part one of this book. So my goal is to help each client see their body as a resource and a place that feels like home.

Before we dive deeper into this process of bodyfulness, start by asking yourself these questions:

Have I been paying attention to my body lately?

How is my body communicating to me right now? What is it saying (think sensations, muscles, body temperature, breath, digestion, hunger, thirst . . .)?

Do I accept what it's telling me? In other words, do I trust my body's messages as valid? Or do I tend to ignore them? If so, why do I think that is?

Take the "Bodyfulness Quiz" at the end of the book to get a baseline measure of your current relationship with your body as a resource for healing.

The body is the ultimate truth-teller and it doesn't like to be taken advantage of, used, abused, or ignored. Can you blame it? As the psychiatrist Bessel van der Kolk warns, your body "keeps the score" on everything it experiences—and the body always wins, no matter how much you *do* use, abuse, or ignore it.[2] If you don't pay attention to what it's telling you, your body will get louder; panic attacks, migraines, and ulcers can be examples of your body stomping its foot and screaming like an ignored child.

How can the body hold the key to your well-being when it seems like your mind is the place where you experience joys, sorrows, worries, and pleasure? It's complicated and somewhat confusing, so I'll boil it down to three things: First, the body absorbs and stores all past experiences, which are expressed through things such as bodily sensations, your nervous system, and muscles, to name a few. Second, the body has its own filtering and recalibration methods, which can be encouraged with certain movements, sounds, and meditations that promote emotional release. These activities release old wounds, which can start to free you from the imbalances they created. They also balance the nervous system and help your different systems flow freely instead of getting lodged. Third, the body is designed to know how you are suffering, where that suffering is showing up, and how to resolve it. *The body's responses are a form of intelligence.* The problem, of course, is that our mind gets in the way. Doubts, distractions, "shoulds," and overanalyzing prevent many people from letting their body do its job. Once people get out of their own way, they can better reconnect to their body's wisdom and healing capacity.

Try to remember the times when your body helped you heal. Start with recalling the last time you were physically sick. What helped your body recover? When was the last time you had an injury? What helped it to heal? When is the last time your body expressed strength of any kind? Expressed joy? How did you know it in your body?

EMBODIMENT AND BODYFULNESS

Bodyfulness is both a set of practices and a lifestyle philosophy I've developed to help my clients get to the root of their discontent—and begin to reconnect with their ease and resiliency. It started with my own lived experiences as I noticed the ways my body helped me feel better when I followed through with what it needed for rest, food, movement, connection, and kindness.

Bodyfulness develops by alternating between your felt-sense, visceral, physical experiences and the mental associations you have of those experiences (embodiment). Embodiment is generally defined as the tangible form of an idea about the body. As Christine Caldwell, the somatic counselor and a fellow pioneer of the word *bodyfulness*, explains it, "Although the body is tangible, and it likely comes from an idea, bodyfulness is more than embodiment; it's cultivated by intentional activities that flow from felt-experience to embodiment . . . the way the body actually oscillates, between top-down and bottom-up processing, the balance between them is what promotes health and well-being."[3] I'll share more of the science behind bodyfulness in the next chapter. For now, think of the concept of *embodiment* as what you see in your mind's eye when you experience something in your body and how you label it mentally, while *bodyfulness* is how it is understood and expressed at the visceral level.

I've woven together existing and emerging healing practices to create my program of bodyfulness. It's a mixture of mindfulness, the latest research on the role of interoception (deep body intelligence), body-based therapies, and a sprinkling of tantra—the ancient philosophy that celebrates the body and the sacred intimacy people share with each other. I'll show you how to incorporate this deeper layer of body wisdom in three progressive stages: embodying mindfulness; developing practices to physically release (or contain at times) older traumas as well as real-time stress; and then ultimately trusting and celebrating your inner confidence and beauty. Think of it as the three *D*s of bodyfulness: diving in, discharging, and delighting!

Mindfulness is currently defined as the awareness that arises through paying attention on purpose, in the present moment and nonjudgmentally, to the unfolding of experience moment by moment.[4]

THE FIRST STAGE: *DIVING* INTO EMBODIED MINDFULNESS

Listening is a skill that comes naturally to some people, while others have to work at it. Me? I have to work at it—in my personal life anyway, whereas talking and expressing myself comes maybe a little too naturally! Whichever camp you fall into, bodyfulness starts with diving into your body's ecosystem and hearing what it has to say. Like all humans, you are most aware of your body during pain, exercise, and sex, but that still leaves a lot of time throughout your life to ignore it. Here, you focus on noticing *what* to pay attention to and then in the second stage you learn *how* to respond to what it's telling you. By listening to the *emergent* or arising whisperings of your body you can prevent *emergencies* from arising unexpectedly later.

> If you listen to your body whisper, you never have to hear it scream.
> —*Unknown*

The good news is you've been listening to the whisperings of your body in one form or another your whole life. Obvious examples include eating when you're hungry and drinking when you're thirsty. Now, whether you satisfy it with a Big Mac and a Coke or a Greek salad and a seltzer water is another matter. There are less overt ways your body talks to you as well—such as when it wants your energy to be balanced and says "I'm sleepy" with a yawn or "Let's blow off some steam" with a sigh. But if you aren't tuned in to what your body is saying, you'll probably miss the balancing cues that it's giving you—unless they get loud and clear, such as eye twitching or a stomachache. But much of the time people tune out those signals or become selective about what they hear, following through only when it's convenient. Some examples of this first stage include noticing:

- what provokes or calms each of your senses and how that relates to your emotions, such as textures that soothe you or music that enlivens you
- an emotion and then tracking its location in your body
- the variations in your breath (deep and full or constricted and choppy) and how they correspond with your mood—for example, it might be difficult to take a full inhale when you're anxious or you may forget to breathe much at all when you're busy
- every time you have pasta you get sleepy or eat pineapple your throat gets scratchy
- your stomach and jaw tense together when you're overthinking
- you feel shame sitting in your belly

Cultivating embodied mindfulness means you're getting savvy at listening to and interpreting your body's language. Decoding its signals can be like learning a new language—you need time and practice to get fluent, to be able to translate regional dialects and slang so you know what each bodily system has to say to *you*. For example, your gut chats in a different way than your diaphragm, your reproductive organs operate unlike your lungs, and your head has different yearnings than your heart. And let's not forget noticing different types of arousal patterns—your "accelerator" compared to your "brakes"—which will come in handy when I talk about physical intimacy and erotic pleasure.

This stage is so healing because it's about relearning how to live in the here and now. Sure, you could say, "But I am in the here and now, stuck in the here and now of my looping, distressed thoughts!" Embodied mindfulness is about listening through the sensory and visceral channels, which you can better trust compared to the ways our brain can fool us by trying to fill in the blanks when we don't have answers. This stage is also powerful because it slows down the emotional chain reaction that can happen instantaneously whenever we're confronted by things that surprise us, put us on guard, or generally cause us to be reactive or impulsive. This is captured beautifully by the psychologist Viktor Frankl, "Between stimulus and response there is space. In that space is our power to choose our response. In our response lies our growth and freedom." Slowing down and noticing our reactive emotional patterns can help us change them and prevent them from being overwhelming to ourselves and others.

Each day, set the intention to notice moments when you're *in* your body and moments when you space out, lost in your thoughts for long periods of time, barely moving or noticing your body.

Here are more examples of *what* to pay attention to before we move on to *how* you handle the messages you do notice (this is by no means an exhaustive list):

Muscles when activated
Muscles when resting
How you're breathing
Posture
Fidgeting or being still

Body temperature
Heaviness in any area
Stiffness or tension in any area
Thirst
Hunger
Fullness
Emptiness
Twitching
Patterns in fatigue
Patterns in energy
Congestion
Which foods digest well
Which food don't digest well
The differences between one side of the body
    and the other
Smells you like and smells you don't like
Times of day you're most present
How laughter feels in your body
How crying feels in your body
Where in your body you feel each of your emotions
The difference between the sensation of pain and the
    sensation of muscles releasing

You could even start by keeping a log of your sleeping, eating, energy, and movement habits. All this information helps you see patterns that work and those that don't work for your mind-body system. Check in a few times a day with your emotional state and where you notice those emotions are located within your body.

If you're not used to being in your body, be patient as you discover these nuances; it will likely be a steep learning curve as you get more comfortable with the uncomfortable. This is a time to tend and befriend yourself, as I discussed in the last chapter. Practice oscillating your attention from within your body to outside of your body. Slow, intentional practices—yoga, tai chi, walking, and breathing techniques—can be ideal for listening within because they help you let go of *thinking* in order to be *sensing*. This doesn't mean you can't be curious about the dynamics of your body while you're skydiving or going down a waterslide, but you're obviously more likely to be distracted by other stimulation and subsequent reactions. Either way, expect that you *will* get distracted, especially if this is a new practice for you. It's normal for the mind to meander with random thoughts as soon as it gets uncomfortable to be in the body. This can vary from person to person, of course, or even from day to day. Honor whatever you need to do to feel safe. As I learned when training with the trauma-sensitive yoga teacher David Emerson, two of the best ways you can come back to the present moment are to notice your breath and notice the dynamics of your muscles as you move them. Thank you, David, you have converted me to believe in this as a credible life hack!

We have to walk before we can run. So, if you're not used to being in your body, it's important to take things slow. Start with one body part at a time; listen to its messages and move on to the next. Examples of things you can do: Blink your eyes a couple times. Wiggle your fingers and toes. Move an arm, leg, hip, or hand, one at a time. Start labeling how these movements feel with basic words such as *tight, stiff, loose, cracking, smooth, pulsing*. Add in adjectives such as *hot, cold, watery, heavy*. Notice how outside factors influence your inner bodily experience and vice versa. The moment you begin to feel uncomfortable in your body, notice what you can do to soothe yourself. It can take some practice to adjust to this inner landscape. As is the case with many things that are worthwhile, you may feel some discomfort before you feel better. Most transformative changes are slow.

THE SECOND STAGE:
DISCHARGING AND RELEASE

One of my clients told me she'd been practicing "sitting with her feelings," as her mindfulness teacher had suggested. She came to

> The body is not the only thing we work with, but it's the only thing we can get our hands on.
> —Ida Rolf

me with a valid question: "And now what?" This part of bodyfulness is more than paying attention on purpose, more than noticing cause and effect. It's knowing what to *do* with what you've paid attention to. Cultivating tools to regulate yourself with dynamic movement is where bodyfulness begins to diverge from mindfulness.

I love the saying "The only way out is through," and that's what this step is about. All emotions in our body are different types of energy that want acknowledgment and then want to move on (e-motion, energy in motion). Bodyfulness is the practice of learning how to recognize and release these energies, especially the stressful ones, so your whole being can learn from them and recalibrate. Put more bluntly: use it or lose it. Research agrees: when people sit less and move more they live longer.[5]

This is where I suggest clients develop a toolbox of releasing methods that fit the emotional experience they're having. For every emotion and corresponding feeling you have, let there be a corresponding movement. Aim to have a variety of activities throughout your week that are a mix of strengthening and soothing, slow and fast, indoor and outdoor, heating up (such as cardiovascular movement) and cooling down (such as stretching). This helps keep your body balanced and gives you more options to discharge stress from your body. Plus, then you aren't limited to a gym or a bike because you have enough options within you wherever you go, whether it be a transatlantic flight or cheap motel. Examples of this step include things typically viewed as "exercise," such as:

Stretching, yoga

Repetitive motion activities such as running, biking, swimming, hiking, Nordic skiing

Strength activities such as weights, squats, lunges, core activities

Different types of dancing

And includes physical release not considered exercise, such as:

Rocking

Sweating

Crying

Auditory release such as grunting, sighing, singing, chanting, humming

Yawning

Shaking

Bouncing

And also includes therapeutic bodywork, such as:

Massage

Foam roller

Acupuncture

Breathing activities

Chiropractor

Moving in an aerial silk

Energy work like chakra balancing and Reiki

Notice the difference between deep sensation as it releases from your body versus the sensation of pain. This is not a time to apply the "no pain no gain" motto. If there is outright pain, back off. If it's deep sensation, practice *titration*—a somatic therapy method where you dial things up just a little bit each time. Some people may need to come out of movements after a few breaths, while others might feel comfortable enough to go deeper into their connective tissue before stopping. Think of this release as disease-states leaving your body.

In this second stage, your aim is to let go of stress from your body to bring yourself into balance. It's about developing an interplay with your mind and body where you know how to pay attention, what to pay attention to, and then what to do about it physically. Which is reassuring and empowering! Explore different movements to see what agrees with your body. Getting into the groove of these two stages is how body acceptance and trust begins.

Do you find that you struggle to release from your body—whether it be emotions, movements, or sounds? Some people become masters of constriction due to messages they've received, being blocked by chronic stress, or past trauma. If so, you could start to unblock yourself by letting out long sighs and releasing your jaw after completing a hard task, shaking out your hands and rolling back your shoulders several times after computer use, watching a tearjerker or even eating a hot pepper to induce tears. I once got two parking tickets in the same week and, boy, I had no problem releasing agitation upon seeing that second one on my windshield. I wouldn't recommend that method since there are cheaper ways to break the seal. Channel your inner bodybuilder the next time you work out or when you notice mounting angst within you by letting out loud groans and guttural sounds. Who cares what other people think! It might inspire them to let go with auditory release as well.

Here's the catch: although movement is often the name of the game in this stage, at times you might find that super slow or nonmoving meditations, soothing activities such as a bath or sauna, or even sleeping is what you need. And sometimes instead of movement you will need to practice *containment* in your body to center yourself and prevent intense emotions from spiraling. Containment is the capacity to stay present and hold your emotions within you, so they don't overwhelm you or someone else. Sometimes what life throws at us is just too much to assimilate or release, so we need to pause and go inward for a bit. The somatic therapist Gwen Mc Hale states, "We need enough containment to provide banks to the river of our expression so we can stay in relationship to our experience, to ourselves, and not get washed away in the suffering."[6] Containment is a way to nurture yourself, like a baby being cradled. It creates boundaries between the outside world and your sensory and emotional response. Examples of containment include: wrapping your arms around yourself; curling into a little ball; putting your hands in your armpits; entering a small, dark space; coming into a Child's pose; running your hands up and down the outsides of your legs from your ankles to your hips; placing both hands at your center (your heart and stomach); using a weighted blanket; and having someone else hug you. Experiment to figure out what emotional moments are best handled with some containment before release, or release and then containment.

For some people, being in their body might trigger past trauma. Most of my training in body-centered therapy methods stems from trauma research and practices. Although I'll cover this connection more in the next chapter, it still won't be a comprehensive manual on how to establish safety in your body after complex trauma. There are lots of layers involved in recovering from the impact of trauma, which goes beyond the scope of this book. This is why I've included resources at the back of the book to help you establish safety in your body first, which is essential before embarking on a bodyful path with greater capacity for intimacy.

It's even common for words such as *exercise* and *yoga* to bring up a host of triggering associations. For example, some people recovering from eating disorders and exercise addiction find the idea of prescribed movement provoking. This was the case with my client Kim, a single woman in her thirties who came to me wanting to stop binging and purging and manage her moods. One of our goals was to let go of rigid, all-or-nothing thinking around her eating and exercise habits. Even though I would specifically use the words *movement, body connection,* and *physical release,* what she heard was *exercise.* So she was resistant to my ideas because she didn't want to be compulsive about burning calories and freak out if she missed a day of movement.

After working together for about six months, we had to switch to video sessions due to the COVID-19 pandemic. A few weeks into her social distancing at home, and free from her regular schedule, she began delving into her creative side. Kim was admittedly someone who cared a lot about her appearance, being on trend, and getting attention from men. Now that the pressure was off to attend parties, go to an office, or engage in online dating, she felt a little breathing room to play around, literally. For the first time, she was being more playful in her body, doing things such as wearing old costumes just for the hell of it and dancing in her living room. Inspired by her imagination and the bodyful methods we talked about, her movement routine became more creative. She showed me the flowing stretches she was experimenting with and how they helped her feel more connected to her body. She also started to practice Ayurvedic medicine, an ancient science focused on healthy lifestyle habits (which we'll discuss in chapter 9). All of this helped Kim reframe the word *movement* to mean something more expansive than merely exercise and burning calories. Over time, she felt freedom to move her body in diverse ways because she craved it naturally, not because she was punishing herself for what she'd eaten.

THE THIRD STAGE: *DELIGHT*, INNER CONFIDENCE, AND BEAUTY

The second stage of bodyfulness focused on gathering tools for physical release or containment. This third stage is about savoring what you've built from those tools. You've developed more confidence in your ability to stay regulated through the ups and downs of life, giving you more energy for things beyond survival and the status quo, such as delight and sensuality. At this stage, you engage it in ways that suit you rather than performing

> This very body that we have that's sitting right here right now, with its aches and its pleasures, is exactly what we need to be fully human, fully awake, and fully alive.
> —*Pema Chödrön*

or ascribing to how others or the system thinks you "should" be. This stage is less about your *method* (what you do) and more about your *approach* (your attitude)—to yourself and your lifestyle.

At this point, you've learned how to hear your inner body wisdom. You're plugged into yourself, whether you're taking a walk in the woods or presenting at work. You let yourself sing in the shower, dance at the kitchen sink, and cry with compassion. Free from cultural and historical value judgments, you give yourself permission to take care of yourself and enjoy yourself. These pleasures help make your behaviors intrinsic and self-motivated. You're not walking an arbitrary number of steps because a fitness magazine told you to do so but because you enjoy moving and being in your body with the pleasure it provides.

The inner wisdom gained from bodyfulness—that deeper understanding of the wonders of the body and its patterns and language—connects you with the beauty inside yourself. This inner beauty could be tender, as you hug someone you love, or goofy, as you roll down a hill with your child. You find a sense of ease and belonging in your body more often. It can be described as peaceful, empowering, vivacious, exuberant, animated, soft, expressive, energetic, magnetic, enlivened, surrender, sweet, connected, aware, grounded, centered, expansive, awake, exhilarating, alive, pulsating, flowing, and . . . pleasurable. The yoga teacher Stephen Cope talks about this concept: "As we begin to re-experience a visceral reconnection with the needs of our bodies, there is a brand-new capacity to warmly love the self. We experience a new quality of authenticity in our caring, which redirects our attention to our health, our diets, our energy, our time management. This enhanced care for the self arises spontaneously and naturally, not as a response to a 'should.' We are able to experience an immediate and intrinsic pleasure in self-care."[7] As the French say, joie de vivre—a zest for life.

This stage also has a flavor of tantric philosophy, developed from the ancient Vedic tradition into the classical traditions of Hinduism. The word *tantra* literally means "expansion," which emerges from a safe, centered place within you. Naturally I've always been drawn to tantra for its philosophy revering the pleasures and wisdom of the body. I love its focus on melting into the pleasures that are already here, within us and around us, rather than grasping for things elsewhere, especially craving the things we can't have. This wave of bodyfulness channels the tantric idea of bringing sensual awakening to even the tedious or benign moments of life. The Ecstatic Living Institute calls tantra "the weaving of spirituality, love, and intimacy into the fabric of our daily life. Tantra encourages honest, intimate communication in order to be authentic in the passion you share with someone else."[8]

After diving in and then discharging out, we now come to a place of *delighting*; a way to notice gratitude right now in your everyday life rather than what is missing, wrong, needs work, or isn't enough. One caveat: you have to give yourself *permission* to own these embodied experiences, and balanced pleasure as your birthright. Examples of this stage of bodyfulness include:

Trusting your body's messages
Confidence in your ability to self-soothe
Having boundaries with yourself and others
Skill with interrupting loops of overthinking
Being playful, silly
Seeing humor around you, including being able
    to make fun of yourself
Trusting your intuition
Following through on your intuition
Tolerating discomfort in a healthy way
Being less reactive
Feeling present
Celebrating
Taking risks
Going with the flow
Being sensual and erotic
Owning your desire rather than questioning it
Expressing creativity

Being emotionally or physically vulnerable

Loving your body

One of the ways I knew I had made it to this stage of bodyfulness was when I decided to take an Introduction to Burlesque class. Here I had been touting the benefits of doing a variety of movements and singing the praises of dancing, yet I didn't have much dance in my own life. Dancing is like a crossword puzzle for your mind because you engage both sides of your brain doing bilateral movements. I started doing Zumba and hip-hop dance classes and gave zero cares about fumbling in the back row, because I was having fun while also being challenged. Then I decided to try burlesque after I saw a colleague do it. I realized I couldn't just talk the talk about owning our sensuality and pleasures, I needed to walk the talk—or in this case, shimmy, hip grind, and drop it like it's hot. It was such a different, dynamic way to engage with my body, and I loved it. Granted, I only told a select few about my group performance at the end of class but, hey, we're all entitled to discretion. The last section of the book will help you develop this third layer.

HOMECOMING

When you think of home, hopefully you conjure images of a cozy place. Inhabiting the body means there is a sense of belonging that feels like home; it means respecting it and appreciating it. Whereas *using* your body means you're pushing it beyond its limitations too much too often. Being bodyful also means having a relational quality with your body, working together as partners. This idea is captured sweetly by the poet Nayyirah Waheed: "and i said to my body. softly. 'i want to be your friend.' it took a long breath. and replied 'i have been waiting my whole life for this.'"[9] What a soulful reunion it can be to return home to your body after years of disdain.

Body shame has become so rampant in the US that nine out of ten people, when shown a silhouette of their body, have a negative emotional response.[10] My client Sharon remembers as a child watching her mom, who was always on diets, look at herself in the mirror and state, "I'm ugly." Sharon had always seen herself in her mom, like any daughter might do with their primary caregiver, so this crushed her. If her mom always thought she was ugly when she had extra pounds, what did that mean about Sharon's appearance and worth?

The natural pull of your body to keep you thriving doesn't stand a chance if you hold it in contempt. Hating on your body is toxic and tiring, and it impacts your self-worth. So please stop body hating—of yourself and others. All bodies are not treated equally in the US. We live within systems and structures that thrive off our continued body disconnection and shame. Sonya Renee Taylor, the author of *The Body Is Not an Apology*, speaks of the need for radical self-love for ourselves in these bodies as a result of "toxic media messaging, systemic bigotry and inequality, and years of shaming," which have caused "body terrorism."[11] She defines body terrorism as the devastating impacts of body hatred in the forms of physical and psychological attacks on the body. This includes racist, homophobic, and transphobic violence; sexual assault; stigma toward disabled and older bodies; and media messages that incite eating disorders, debilitating shame, and mass self-hatred. Body terrorism clearly creates a barrier to bodyfulness. It's time we stop making the body less valuable than the mind, *and* it's time to stop "othering" bodies oppressively. Everyone loses when we place some bodies as inherently better than others because of their skin color, shape, or performative value.

What if reverence for your body was something you let yourself want and value rather than resist, question, or occasionally dabble with? Write a letter to your body describing how much you adore it. In an act of defiance to all the systems and messages telling you your body is less than, be radically loving in your admiration for your body—*all* of it. Then imagine what your life could feel like if this were your reality.

Although the system has gaslighted us about our bodies, you have the power to disrupt that. Instead of being critical, be curious;

observe your body's messages with wonder and appreciation for the information they offer. Relate to your body in a manner that is more adoring. Have fun in your body, stretching, singing, dancing, or luxuriating in ways that simply feel good. Being able to notice, allow, and enjoy your bodily experiences, both physically and emotionally with respect, is life changing.

~ 7 ~

Our Issues Are
in Our Tissues

> If you cannot feel satisfaction in ordinary everyday
> things like taking a walk, cooking a meal, or playing
> with your kids, life will pass you by.
> —*Bessel van der Kolk*

IT'S COMMON TO BE suspicious of less conventional methods in medicine, to wonder if they're legit with real studies to back them up. For some, the concept of bodyfulness might seem fairly out there, but it's actually an integration of established methods, emerging neuroscience, and intimacy practices, holistically applied to our modern ailments. This is where the future of health is headed.

The science supporting bodyfulness is part of a renaissance within psychotherapy that recognizes the importance of the body to cleanse and cope with emotions. Evidence shows that emotional stress gets trapped in the body in ways the logical mind can't initially process. Bodyfulness is similar to other somatic methods by going straight to the source of that stress in the body to release it. Somatic methods are powerful techniques that help explain and unlock the ways trauma lingers in our bodies. Unlike most somatic methods, bodyfulness goes beyond stress recovery to encourage and provide a roadmap for people to reclaim life's pleasures and joys, seeing them as vital to preventative health. Just as people initially discounted the benefits of mindfulness meditation but now sing its praises, somatic therapies such as bodyfulness are gaining recognition and validity, pivoting the course of treatments from solely talk therapy.

In part one of this book, I discussed the barriers to being bo-dyful from historical and cultural perspectives. Here it gets more individual as I explain the ways your own mind and body can be a dumping ground for these dysfunctions, and how *you* hold the power to recalibrate and recharge yourself. Let's geek out together on the fascinating science underlying bodyfulness.

YOUR NERVOUS SYSTEM, THE CONDUCTOR

The number one job of your brain-body system is always to keep you safe. Together the brain—the physical place where the inner-workings of our mind percolate—and the body respond immediately when you're in danger and clue you in when that danger has passed. How do they keep up with the information coming at you every second of every day? By employing the reticular activation system, your internal "bodyguard" that scientists say helps determine what information is worthy of your attention. If it notices something threatening, or even *similar* to a past threat, it alerts your nervous system, the "conductor" for this orchestra of your body. It keeps you centered and calmly aware, which are both precursors to experiencing pleasure. Or it can literally be a *nervous* system, constantly tense and on guard, armoring your body—the opposite of pleasure.

Your nervous system has three main branches: the *sympathetic*, which controls your fight-flight-freeze response; the *parasympathetic*, which controls your rest-and-digest response; and the *enteric*, which I'll discuss later. The former is the gas pedal in the car, ready to re-spond to perceived dangers. Fight mode is about physical aggression, which can show up as crabby or argumentative behavior. Flight mode is about escaping, which can look like social withdrawal, substance abuse, or TV watching. Freeze mode is the fight-or-flight response on hold, such as when we mentally check out and detach because we feel stuck in the threat. When disconnection from the body is severe it's called *dissociation*, meaning the mind escapes as an attempt to lessen emotional pain. It works in the short term, but when you routinely disregard the body, it will eventually give you some sort of pushback.

On a more pleasant note, think of the parasympathetic's rest-and-digest mode as a pause button or the brakes of your car, which slow you down and chill you out. This state of ease and steadiness can be a springboard for experiencing sensual, playful, lively, and sexual/erotic pleasures, as well as enjoyable and empathic connections with others. There's nothing wrong with having some fight-or-flight activation, of course; stress is motivating and necessary at times. For example, in the workplace we want to hit the flow channel I mentioned in chapter 2, that place where the task is hard enough to make us grow but not so hard that we break down. The problem with stress is how unmanageable and pervasive it can be, robbing us of ease and delight. Which has been the case with America's collective nervous system, so to speak.

Check out the "Language of Sensations Handout" at the end of the book to learn the signs that indicate whether your body feels in fight, flight, freeze, or ease.

TRAUMA AND STRESS, THE THIEVES

Given that "safety first" is your body's motto, physical and emotional harm—real or imagined—obviously get in the way of pleasure and satisfying relationships. And yet the natural state of all mammals is to be on guard. For example, most people's pleasant life experiences become faint memories and their unsavory experiences stick out in their memory. The psychologist Rick Hanson puts it well, saying that we are like Teflon for pleasant moments and Velcro for challenging ones. Anything stressful is written in bold in the catalog of our body and brain as a way to prevent it from happening again. We think, "I'd better not forget or I'll be duped again." This is why past adversity may still haunt you. And why we need to actively seek out things that soothe us or pleasantly excite us to balance out this *negativity bias*.

> Taboo topics are not around us. They are in our nervous system.
> —Ilan Stephani

If the reticular activation system is the bodyguard of information coming in, and the nervous system is the conductor of it all, then trauma and stress are the provocateurs who trigger you, thieves who rob you of security and comfort. Take note that there are important differences between trauma and stress—in severity and in your perception of the experience. Trauma is defined as any experience that overwhelms your ability to cope and respond, and it leaves you feeling helpless and out of control. Whereas with stress you have a sense of control, or at least a modicum of influence, over your situation. Having this sense of internal agency over deciding what you need and what feels best in the moment is important to feeling strong and safe again from those pleasure thieves.

Trauma comes in thirty-two flavors. Most people think of trauma as a specific event that shocked the body, like the impact to a war veteran, rape victim, or car accident survivor. The worst kind of trauma, with good reason, is when a person can't move or speak, lacking agency, such as when they're being held down or prematurely coming out of anesthesia. This is the most traumatizing to your body compared to when you can move—run away or verbally and physically defend yourself—times when you can practice agency. Even smaller traumas happen to people all the time, and these microaggressions can accumulate inside your nervous system.

You may hear the word *trauma* and think, "That's not something I've dealt with." But the likelihood is you have; we all have. Research is recognizing traumas stemming from early childhood relationships, such as neglect, abandonment, or even mixed messages. The percentage of people with some unresolved adverse childhood experiences (ACEs)—including problems with attachment to caregivers or other developmental, cultural, and intergenerational traumas—make almost everyone a member of the Trauma Club.

Yes, even hard shit that happened to your parents and grandparents before you were born is inherited and influences your temperament, sense of self, and relationship style. Intergenerational trauma stems from family suffering, such as a loss, like the death of an infant, or from societal trauma such as slavery and genocide. Science is only beginning to understand this world of epigenetics, but we do know that trauma leaves a chemical mark on a person's genes, changing the way it's expressed, which is passed down to subsequent generations. The psychologist Carl Jung said, "Nothing has a stronger influence psychologically on their environment and especially on their children than the unlived life of the parent."[1]

In my case, my parents' upbringing as essentially orphans was a factor in leading me to inherit a feeling of abandonment insecurities and a desire to resolve them—at least once I realized how much they affected my relationship patterns! My mom's mother died giving birth to her, and she bounced from relative to relative before being sent to her dad in high school. She hated it so much that, after getting permission to visit a cousin for the weekend, she hopped on a Greyhound bus with a secret plan to never return. My dad's father died suddenly when he was seven, leaving his mother a widow with three small boys. Too much for her to manage, he was raised in a foster home. I have no doubt my parents' experiences influenced my professional decision to focus on relationships as a way to heal and temper my own epigenetic blueprint and help prevent others from feeling "separate."

Fortunately, although trauma may be passed on to us, we can modulate the legacy we're given by learning to embody our inherent right to ease and connection. Rev. angel Kyodo williams puts it beautifully: "We also carry all the joy and the laughter. . . . Our history did not begin with us being stolen off the African continent . . . in my bones, in my blood, in my body, I know what it is to be free, this isn't a thing I need to imagine this is a thing I need to remember."[2]

This chapter is meant to give you a general understanding of what causes more mild forms of disembodiment. If you have experienced deep trauma injuries that are unresolved, I recommend you work with a qualified trauma therapist so that you create a strong container to support you on your healing journey. There are some excellent books focusing on complex trauma that I include in my Trauma Resource Guide at the end of the book.

BODY MEMORY

It was recently estimated that 60 percent of physical medical problems are emotionally induced.[3] And where do our emotions originate? In our body. The physical body reflects the truth of our history and our emotional experiences.[4] And yet how exactly are memories and intergenerational injuries stored in our body? Well, we know that our brain stores mental memories (in the hippocampus), and we know we have muscle memory (kinesthetic memory), like when we improve at tennis or the piano. But we also have emotional memory from trauma or stress, traces left inside our cells and tissues like a phantom or something undigested. This stress, before (in utero) and during our lifetime, gets lodged in our nervous system if we don't have ways to move it out of us. For example, one of my clients had a car accident years ago when someone didn't stop at a stop sign, hitting her from the right side. For months, whenever she came to a similar four-way intersection she would flinch if she saw a car coming from her right. Over time, whenever this scenario presented itself she would take full breaths to calm her nervous system and muscles, then reposition and reorient herself to the present as a way to override this past body memory.

Bessel van der Kolk, a psychiatrist and the author of the seminal somatic therapy book *The Body Keeps the Score*, suggests that we have maps of ourselves in the world encoded in the visceral part of ourselves—the organs of our chest, abdomen, and pelvis.[5] This emotional body memory is a type of nonverbal language, and sometimes that language is living out our *past* trauma; we can tell by the way we might react disproportionately to what is happening. As the counselor Wendy Kritzer stated, "All emotions, even those that are suppressed and unexpressed, have physical effects. Unexpressed emotions tend to stay in the body like small ticking time bombs—they are illnesses in incubation."[6]

In his book *Waking the Tiger*, the psychologist Peter Levine explains that "traumatic symptoms are not caused by the 'triggering' event itself. They stem from the frozen residue of energy that had not been resolved or discharged; this residue remains trapped in the nervous system where it can wreak havoc on our bodies and spirits."[7] In chapter 9 I'll discuss this concept of body energy and specific activities to balance it in different areas of your body.

Healing comes from acknowledging and "digesting" past trauma memories. This is done by overriding past experience of helplessness and creating new associations of strength within your body with your agency—the opportunity for choices and taking action. With agency you don't feel stuck, you're able to engage with stimuli as needed to change your situation and feel safe again. The second stage of bodyfulness is a way to practice having agency. Over time, this leads to the third stage of bodyfulness, developing body trust and being able to let go. This ability to tolerate vulnerability because you know you can handle it by taking actions to stabilize yourself is one mighty superpower.

What are a couple activities that typically help you feel calmer? Where and how do you start to feel that calm in your body? What are a couple activities that typically help you feel more alert? Where and how do you tend to feel that in your body?

THE REGULATOR

When you regularly balance your nervous system with agency, whether it be with breathing and moving or seeking rest and containment, it becomes more *regulated*. This leads to stress relief, better sleep and digestion, boosted immunity, better energy levels, and as I'll explain in the next chapter, the ability to *co-regulate* harmoniously with others. Being able to regulate your nervous system is a way to be adaptive rather than reactive to your experiences. Being regulated doesn't mean your nervous system is always in one particular state; it means you have the capacity to be flexible and move through different states, eventually returning to a place of composure, that home base of safety and security.

Bodyful practices help people feel regulated by teaching them to use their body as a resource to discharge the old stress and practice new ways to feel safe, present, empowered, and connected to the outside world in a pleasant way. Examples of a regulated brain-body system include welcoming the types of pleasure I shared in chapter 2—sensual, playful, liveliness, and erotic/sexual—as well as altruistic behaviors and coping with relationship challenges. Some examples of an unregulated brain-body system would be addictions, eating disorders, anxiety, depression, a general lack of vitality, isolating, and constant fighting, among others.

THE SCIENCE OF STAGE ONE: EMBODIED MINDFULNESS

The Western medical model long thought that talking and mental analyzing alone could control this built-up body angst. We now know managing bodily emotions actually helps inform our mental logic as well. For all my praise about the body's wisdom, I definitely believe that engaging in dialogue can be tremendously healing; not all talk is cheap—expressing and sharing verbally can increase clarity, connection, and trust. My beef is that focusing on the mind without the body is like a couple going to therapy and only one person doing the talking. How the heck will improvements occur when half the equation is MIA?

Let me break this down with neuroscience to explain why leaving out the body, and only trying to talk or think about past pain, is limiting. For starters, memory retrieval and language become compromised when there's been trauma.

- Broca's area, in the left hemisphere of the brain, is responsible for speech production. During trauma, blood flow is limited to this area. When a person with post-traumatic stress is reminded of their traumatizing event visually or verbally, Broca's area shuts down and the person can't integrate the trauma memory into a narrative.[8] Deep, guttural sounds such as sighing or groaning can vibrate and help release their viscera (emotional body memory). This is why I suggest clients engage in auditory release to discharge stress and balance themselves.

- The amygdala is the part of the brain that attaches emotional significance to memories, making strong emotions such as fear and shame or even joy and love hard to forget. When we are in a scary situation, the amygdala directs where our attention goes. It may zone in on a detail of the experience, such as the grip of a hand on our neck, or direct attention away from what's happening toward meaningless details. What gets attention most often are fragmented bodily sensations, so that is usually what becomes encoded into our memory. And why working with sensations is helpful because you're going straight to the source of the original injury.
- The prefrontal cortex is the part of our brain responsible for choosing what to focus on, such as rational thought and impulse control. It becomes impaired, and often even shuts down, when there is a surge of stress hormones. When this happens, it's much harder to control what we pay attention to and to make sense of what we are experiencing. So later on, we are less able to remember our experience in an orderly way or apply logic to confront traumatic memories.
- The hippocampus encodes our experiences into short-term memory and stores them as long-term memories. Fear impairs its ability to encode and store "contextual information," such as the layout of the room where something scary happened. Fear also impairs its ability to encode time-sequencing information.

The relationship between the amygdala and hippocampus is like a dance between implicit memory (emotional/unconscious memory) and explicit memory (the ability to form *new* memories). The amygdala feeds on repeated fear, and stress strengthens and increases its neurons. At the same time, fear and stress decrease hippocampus neurons. This makes it difficult to form new memories without the taint of old ones. An overactive amygdala plus a shrunken hippocampus means that we can have painful experiences in our unconscious memory without any current memory of them.

When a therapist or friend says "Tell me what happened," it can make a person stammer trying to explain the details. And it's no wonder. Some parts of them had checked out, whereas some parts had gone on high alert. Either way, somatic practices such as bodyfulness reorient these areas of the brain I just mentioned by starting at the source, in the body where the trauma got stuck to begin with. This is why the first stage of bodyfulness is so important. It's a direct way to practice listening to your body on a visceral level, in order to notice what's there and then experiment with how to let it go and release these old imprints.

What about Mindfulness?

You might be wondering, "But doesn't mindfulness already do that?" It certainly helps, which is why embodied mindfulness is the first stage of bodyfulness. The practice of paying attention to what you're experiencing as it is happening and the emotions and subsequent feelings that arise, all without judgment, helps you mentally understand your responses and reactions. For example, have you ever had a conversation with someone that left you feeling frustrated, only to take your frustration out on someone else later? Mindfulness can help you notice that, and maybe even help you understand why the initial conversation made you feel that way and how your feelings colored the second conversation. *But then what?*

Mindfulness is an important first step, but it's not enough. Although it helps us notice cause and effect, it lacks two crucial next steps: physically discharging the reactivity within our nervous system patterns and visceral body, and building agency (which comes from those actions we chose). If you want to change your reactive behaviors, you need to do more than analyze them. Taking physiological action leads to change, not merely thinking about acting.

I get why mindfulness is all the rage these days—there's mindful everything: mindful hair care, mindful business conferences, mindful jewelry. There's even "Mindfulness-based Mind Fitness Training" where the word mind is listed not once but twice! But it is more than a marketing buzzword. It's a critical component in learning how to change neural pathways in your brain, especially when it doesn't stray too far from its Buddhist roots. Plus, there has been a boom of research in recent decades looking at the benefits of mindfulness when it's practiced regularly as meditation. Its potential benefits—including mental clarity, reduced reactivity, and increased compassion for yourself and others—are what led me to incorporate mindfulness into my work with clients as the first step to cultivating body connection.[9]

Although several studies find that a person's ability to be mindful can help them better handle the stress of relationship conflict and express themselves in social situations, other research shows that it can be modestly helpful, at best, in reducing anxiety, depression, and pain.[10] Here's the thing: mindful practices *are* limited because, as emerging research shows, *our issues are in our tissues.* We may be thinking, obsessing, and worrying about our "issues," but our issues and the effects of our obsessing also become lodged quite literally in our connective tissue called *fascia* (the neurofascial system). The body holds on to anything it can't let go of or digest—unprocessed emotions, trauma, stress—which begins to manifest as physical and emotional dis-ease and eventually becomes full-on disease. So while mindfulness has several benefits, certainly in the short term, it's still a practice that keeps the focus in our head, and keeps us thinking about our body but not acting, releasing, and rewiring the past stress that lives in the body.

There are also people who find being quiet and still pretty threatening. They may be scared of being focused on their body and would benefit from easing into mindfulness or any still meditation. This is why I specifically tailor the order of embodied mindfulness and then movement (or vice versa) according to my clients' level of trauma.

Interoceptive Awareness

Engaging experimentally with your body can help you put the pieces together about your reactive patterns in order to change them. This builds keen body intelligence, called *interoception*. For example, when some of my clients first start practicing yoga regularly, they report that a steady wave of changes takes place within, such as more awareness of their breath, muscles, and digestion. That made sense to them, but they'd be perplexed about why moving their body into pretzel-like positions helped them feel more clarity, less on edge, and more confident.

Research studying interoception, nuanced awareness for internal body states, is trying to explain this. It is increasingly being recognized as the eighth sense, along with sight, sound, smell, taste, and touch (which I'll discuss in chapter 10), as well as vestibular sense (balance) and proprioceptive sense.

When we have proprioception, we know where our body is as it moves in space, such as knowing where our feet go as we walk, even though we're not looking down at them. Interoceptive awareness is the internal version of this. There isn't one place within you to pinpoint interoception but rather a series of interacting systems throughout the body. With interoception, you recognize the moment-by-moment changes of your inner states—sensations; emotions; circulation; different physiological systems such as the cardiorespiratory system (breathing), gastrointestinal (digesting) system, nociceptive system (pain), endocrine (hormone) and immune (illness) systems—so you can figure out your needs and resolve them. Talk about being dialed in!

Just like other sensory systems, the interoceptive system has special receptors located throughout the body. These receptors in our organs, skin, and muscles deliver information through the nervous system to the insular cortex, our receiving zone that reads the physiological state of the entire body and then generates emotions, such as hunger and craving, which bring about actions to keep the body in a state of internal balance.[11] When the brain integrates these sensory experiences, it puts them together to come up with an emotional assessment. As an example, if you notice your breathing is shallow, your heartbeat is fast, and you have the jitters, you're likely to assess that you're nervous.

Through your interpretation, the brain then organizes systems to respond to your changing inner conditions. Motor pathways communicate from the brain to the body to change behavior in order to feel better within. The brain evaluates the interoceptive information, categorizes and connects it with other sensory information, and stores the associations in memory. In this way, we learn awareness and strategies to maintain emotional and physical stability again in the future, which is important for overall well-being.

It's hypothesized that some mental health problems are due to problems of interoception, meaning something is off when it comes to the person's ability to connect with the network of systems in their body moment by moment, sense by sense. Science is now finding that focusing on bodily awareness and movement is a powerful intervention for problems of self-regulation, such as eating disorders and substance abuse.[12] Medicine had told us that these problems are biochemical or genetic disorders—things you can't change or can only be controlled by medication. But now they are being understood as things we have influence over with interoception.

I see interoception as the process that bridges all layers of bodyfulness. This rich understanding of cause and effect in your body and mind helps you reclaim body trust, a type of implicit knowing. Whether you're trying to overcome trauma or just navigate your day in a harried world, being able to trust your body is huge. From body trust you feel more wisdom and confidence, freeing you up to experience moments of pleasure, big and small.

THE SCIENCE OF STAGE TWO: MOVEMENT IS MEDICINE

My client Leila told me, "I know in my head what I should do but I don't know why I don't live it." Just because you understand the source of an impulse or behavior, or mentally understand why you feel a certain way, doesn't mean you know *how* to change the emotion or behavior. So after mindfully listening in the first stage of bodyfulness, we must somehow physically release or actively discharge the energy of stress from the whole body, not only the cells and connective tissues but also the digestive, musculoskeletal, lymphatic, and nervous systems. That "somehow" happens when we include the body in the process; when we move the mind's attention into the body and employ a variety of techniques tailored to its particular needs—when we practice bodyfulness.

People don't always have the words or wherewithal to express themselves. Yet when they engage in physical activity, things click and they get a burst of aha! I once took an overnight flight to Australia. Hours of squirming, not nearly enough water, and three romantic comedies later, I arrived in a mental fog. When I made it to my hotel and saw that big bed with crisp white sheets it was like the heavens parted. Except that it was 1 p.m. and sunny. My body hadn't realized I was on a different hemisphere. My spine ached, my eyelids were heavy, and my breath . . . full-on halitosis. But rather than nap, I dragged myself to a nearby park for a brisk walk. In that hour I was revived.

What happened? I made myself move and my body worked its magic. An abundance of studies—too many to even try to include them all—confirm that when people exercise they feel better and live longer. As someone who's identified as an athlete just about longer than anything else, it comes as no surprise. Some of my biggest moments of clarity and most genuine conversations have happened during these outdoor endeavors. I see this with my clients when we have sessions where we walk and talk. Put people in the outdoors with their hearts pumping and things start flowing.

Make America Breathe Again

What happens when we engage in movement, whether it be of the mellow variety or more vigorous? For starters, we engage the breath.

A healthy mind has an easy breath.
—*Unknown*

One of the best ways to stay steady in this unsteady world is with the breath. It is a beautiful bridge between the body and mind. Now, obviously you breathe every day, but are you barely breathing your way through life? When the breath is consistently full and rhythmic, like an ocean wave, you can take full advantage of the benefits it offers. I always tell my clients, "No breath is wasted." Your next breaths set in motion a ripple effect of changes—everything from getting blood flowing to helping rinse out toxins to balancing your mood and stress levels.

Think you need to set aside a bunch of time for exercise? Even five minutes can make a difference. Start one breath at a time. Unlike digestion and other systems of the body, the breath is something we have control over. And given it helps us regulate our internal body states, it seems too good to be true! Try to not overlook it.

Research shows that long, full breaths, especially long exhalations that release into the abdomen, help engage the rest-and-digest mode and stimulate the following body functions: saliva production, digestion, sexual arousal, crying, urination, and defecation. Whereas sweating, goose bumps, dilated pupils, raised blood pressure, constipation, a relaxed bladder (yes, peeing your pants), and the inability to get an erection or vaginal lubrication are examples of the fight-flight-freeze mode.

In addition to exhaling, there are other bodily functions that have releasing benefits, such as sighing, sweating (when it's not a by-product of threat), and crying. Sweat releases toxic chemicals from the body, signals hormonal messages such as stress and attraction, and may be as unique as a fingerprint.[13] And the next time you apologize for crying, keep in mind that it's not a burdensome response; it's self-soothing and cathartic.[14] Tears also show others that we're vulnerable, which is critical to human connection and empathy. Crying even sends emotional signals to reduce sexual arousal in another person.[15]

Move It or Lose It

Sitting is the new smoking, in which case the average American is "smoking" a pack a day. The remedy? Move. The neuroscientist

Wendy Suzuki's TED talk cited moving your body as the number one most transformative thing you can do right now.[16] Why? Because it has immediate effects on your body and brain. Exercise increases the feel-good neurotransmitters of dopamine, serotonin, endorphins, and norepinephrine in your brain, as well as *enkephalins* that help with a sense of well-being. A single workout improves focus and re-action times for up to two hours. With regularity, you can have long-term effects on the function of the brain. It's like a muscle: the more you work out, the less aging and fogginess of the brain. The key is getting your heart rate up and doing at least thirty minutes at a time.

The holistic psychiatrist Henry Emmons states that "getting regular vigorous exercise is the best possible way that you can alter your own brain chemistry and improve your mood."[17] As Emmons explains, scientifically we're understanding what actually happens as a result of "feeling the burn" of exercise: increased body tempera-ture can lead to a more relaxed state; deep breathing can help with oxygen flow and oxygenation of the brain and other vital organs and clear toxins from your system. Emotional benefits of exercise include helping to alleviate stress, anxiety, and depression; improve self-confidence, and if it's done with others, increase compassion and connection. Exercise really is a wonder drug.

If you don't have different ways to move and release, a neuromus-cular pattern of bodily contraction develops. The psychologist Peter Levine has studied the stress response by observing both animals and people. He explains that animals engage in the adaptive act of shuddering or shaking off stress to release stuck fight-flight-freeze energy.[18] Clearly all animals need to shake off stress, and that includes human animals. This is why bodyfulness encourages vigorous move-ment as a way to "shake" out the past and feel renewed. We have much to learn from the ways animals engage their bodies to release stress. It's part of our survival and evolutionary adaptation.

Let It Flow to Let It Go

Where exactly does stress get stuck inside of us? Although it "lives" in our nervous system as reactivity, it also lands in fascia, our connective tissue. Without fascia you would be a wet noodle on the floor with no form; it's like a maze or spiderweb throughout the body surrounding muscle, bones, nerves, vessels, and organs. If there's restriction in the fascia of your body, you feel some sort of blockage, such as heavy, achy muscles.

The term *neurofascial* describes the connective tissue and the nervous system coming together. Our fascia consists of nerves that detect pain, especially when they're stimulated. Agitation, such as stress, releases neuropeptides into our fascia, which harden the tissue. Fascial "memory" is caused by collagen forming in these areas of stress by the transmission of pain and other impulses released from nerve endings after emotional trauma. This encodes memory traces in the connective tissue. Feeling renewed ease and tissue function has been reported from people who received neurofascial massage.[19]

Science is finding that the psoas muscle is one of the main areas where stress gets stuck in our tissues. The psoas muscle starts at the front of our hips and winds into the abdomen and low back, connecting our torso to our legs. This muscle is responsible for lifting our legs (to run—pretty crucial) and bending forward at the waist. Our psoas activates when the stress response kicks in. It also attaches to and crosses over the diaphragm (the muscle that controls breath, and a reactive emotional center of our body) with connective tissue. If that tissue is constantly tight, it interferes with our breath and sets in motion a chain effect of not having enough blood flow to the brain or digestion. Even more, both the psoas and diaphragm link to the brain stem and spinal cord, considered our primal reactive brain. Quite the emotional powerhouse that psoas! This is why a chronically tight psoas can even exhaust the adrenal glands and deplete the immune system.[20]

Each new triggering event, even a mildly stressful one, has a cumulative effect as the psoas "remembers" what it learned from the original traumatic event. For example, a woman with sexual trauma and a contracted psoas might experience pain during intercourse as a result of the psoas's conditioned, high-alert state. This is why releasing the psoas often brings up old emotions that were stored there.

Use a foam roller or tennis ball to target the fascia, which becomes thick and less elastic from physical and emotional challenges. Experiment with how it feels to roll up and down your spine, and other areas of your back, then move on to your legs. To focus on the psoas, set the foam roller aside and practice lunges, one leg at a time. Keep the knee of your leg extended behind you on the ground to better isolate the psoas, and engage your core muscles so you don't dump pressure into the low back.

Movement Therapies

Science is learning that movement therapies, which help clients connect to interoception, breath, and blood flow, improve the immune system and inflammatory response, the enteric brain in the gut, and release stuck trauma in the sheaths of connective tissue, such as the psoas, in the body.

The kind of breathing done in contemplative movement practices such as yoga, dance, and tai chi helps decrease inflammation and promote a healthy *vagal tone*, which is connected to the vagus nerve.[21] Vagal tone is measured by the fluctuations in heart rate that occur with the breath, referred to as heart rate variability (HRV).[22] HRV is a biomarker that measures how well your body adapts to stress. Higher HRV (greater variability between heart beats) is proving to be a sign that your nervous systems are balanced and your body is capable of adapting and responding to what comes your way to perform your best.

Yoga is the main somatic tool I use in client sessions (as you can imagine, it's tricky to go running, skiing, and biking with my clients). Physical benefits of yoga include: flexibility, strength, balance, and decreased cortisol, the stress hormone.[23] Yoga movements, specifically inversions, or anytime your feet are at the same level or higher than your head, improve cardiovascular health and immune response by draining lymphatic fluid. Because the lymphatic system is a closed pressure system and has one-way valves that keep lymph moving toward the heart, when you turn upside down, the entire lymphatic system is stimulated, thus strengthening your immune, nervous, and endocrine systems. Inversions also stimulate the thyroid and parathyroid glands, which secrete hormones that regulate metabolism.[24]

Yoga can also help reorient people to time. As the trauma-informed yoga teacher David Emerson explains, "One characteristic of trauma is that things don't come to an end. . . . With yoga, we can notice the rhythmical quality of events (postures) beginning, being sustained for a period of time, and finally ending."[25] Even more aggressive movement makes a difference. Research shows that people who engage in strength training report feeling more confident.[26] In conversation with my friend and colleague Mariah Rooney, a facilitator of the program "Trauma Informed Weight Lifting," she explained that, in supportive conditions, strength training has the potential to boost self-trust and reduce isolation. Sure seems like body strength translates to mental strength. But you don't have to be a yogi or a bodybuilder to get moving. You just have to decide to be in your body, be open and curious to how different movements feel, and build tolerance for the fluctuations in your breath and muscles day by day.

Keep in mind that you might physically move with exercise all the time but never connect to your sensuality or build interoception during the experience. You could spend a whole spin class or jog thinking about a snarky comment someone made or the way your butt looks in your leggings. You'd get physical benefits, but it wouldn't be an example of embodiment—you were lost in thought the whole time! Intentional, present-centered, and exploratory movement practices not only encourage interoception but also connection to your sensual self.

~ 8 ~

The Pleasure Principle

IF THE THIRD STAGE of bodyfulness was a bumper sticker it would read, "I learn, love, and delight in my body." Or as one of my clients eloquently said, "For me, pleasure as movement, body connection and awareness . . . is freedom itself." This stage is also where bodyfulness is most distinguished from other somatic practices—by specifically focusing on bringing healthy pleasure into your life after trauma and stress. Bodyfulness bridges somatic theories on trauma with pleasure and joy recovery. Most research on trauma mentions that it blocks people from pleasure and joy, but that's where the discussion fizzles, without much further explanation of how to reclaim it. Their focus is on the complexity of establishing safety and embodiment, with pleasure an assumed byproduct. Yet people need facilitation with reclaiming pleasure as well, to go beyond surviving to thriving. Not (necessarily) because we want to make frolicking our full time job but because it gives us resilience and aids in collective well being.

THE SCIENCE OF STAGE THREE: THE ROOTS OF PLEASURE

What happens in our body and brain to produce pleasure? And what does science say about whether we even *need* pleasure? It turns out that both sensory and relationship pleasures have been key to our species' survival by helping us know how to respond, learn, and adapt, as part of the psychological process of reward.[1] The most obvious example is the "pleasure principle," the concept that humans are wired to avoid pain and seek pleasure, such as when something feels too hot and you pull away to avoid getting burned. The brain even has a "pleasure center," the *medial prefrontal cortex*, which is involved in motivating us to explore and learn. Studies indicate that this center is activated by seeing attractive faces, pictures of loved ones, artwork, erotica, and addictive drug cues.[2]

Charles Darwin studied the evolution of emotions and suggested that all mammals experienced moments of pleasure and displeasure and that they are adaptive responses to situations. Scientists have put pleasure into categories: *fundamental pleasures* include food and sexual pleasures, and *higher-order pleasures* include artistic, music, money, and social connections.[3] But whether you're eating a delicious meal, getting paid, seeing beautiful art, or kissing your sweetheart, to the brain it's all the same. They all register in your brain by secreting the chemicals dopamine (the "reward chemical," part of the pleasure/reward system) and sometimes endorphins (part of the norepinephrine/adrenaline arousal system), both strongly associated with good feelings. Thinking about past pleasures, anticipating future ones, or being in a pleasurable moment each involves the same brain systems.

Some people have a more robust drive for this pleasure/reward system. Dr. Helen Fisher, who has combined years of fMRI research on dopamine and brain function, describes these people as "explorers." Characteristics include a sunny personality, optimism, enthusiasm, energy, seeking pleasurable sensations, curiosity, creativity, impulsivity, an intense focus on new stimuli and easily becoming bored. One benefit is they tend to be very adaptable because they learn quickly. Go get 'em, explorers.[4]

The next time you feel a craving, stop and recognize where you feel it in your body, whether it be for food, the outdoors, sex, or sleep. Rather than impulsively indulging the craving, try to slow down and think about what's really driving it. Is it distraction, habit, or is it related to your fundamental survival needs?

Pleasure Leads to Happiness

Science is finding that pleasure is an important component of happiness. The lack of pleasure, called *anhedonia*, is common in those with depression. Although it's not fully clear why the brain regions necessary for pleasure get disrupted with anhedonia, research does indicate that people aren't able to feel happiness without having moments of pleasure. Scientifically, a way to understand the difference between pleasure and happiness is that pleasure is *liking plus wanting* or yearning, whereas happiness involves *liking without the wanting* or craving, which leads to more contentment.[5] Pleasure is intense, so it's more satisfying; happiness packs less of a punch but is more easily sustained. And remember when I explained in chapter 2 that pleasure is more fleeting than happiness? This is by design; the reward sensations produced by our dopamine pleasure system are brief to prevent us from being so absorbed that we become bait for a predator.

Resilience

Being bodyful helps us stay resilient. Resilience is the ability to recover from setbacks and adapt to challenging circumstances. Adapting is a type of learning, and both pleasure and learning are associated with the pleasure center of the brain.

We are not born with a bottomless pit of resilience. We need to have pleasure practices to cultivate it. Resilience can be strengthened by working toward goals and having a sense of purpose; engaging in activities that you're passionate about is indeed replenishing. But resilience can also increase from simple pleasures in life, such as flow states or moments of humor.[6] One study found that weaving in daily activities to induce comedy and laughter reduced depression and increased joy for participants even months later.[7] Perhaps this is why I justify my aforementioned penchant for Tik Tok during the times I'm limited to getting my humor fix from a screen.

Clearly pleasure and happiness are major motivators for our lives. Since our bodies crave balance first and foremost, they will overcompensate if we've been deprived of pleasure, by doing things such as eating too much chocolate, getting drunk, or texting an ex-boyfriend in an attempt to get attention. This is why we need to have powerful pauses—intentional breaks throughout the day and healthy pleasures scattered throughout the week so we're not depriving ourselves. It gives us *neural relaxation*, which fills up our gas tank so we stay strong and better able to care for ourselves and others as well.

In her book *Pleasure Activism*, the author and activist Adrienne Maree Brown talks about having pleasure as your motivation toward changing the world. I would agree, adding that when we choose actions based on knowing what we *want* (versus *should*), it naturally helps us follow through with actions to get us there. Key questions such as "What makes you come alive in your body?" and "What are you passionate about?" can guide your activism in a world that needs it from you, from all of us. Guide your activism energy from your answers because those will be the pursuits that are sustainable and give you the stamina and resilience you need to fight injustice. Importantly, rather than standing up to oppression alone, band together with others. Sonya Renee Taylor said that the systems are designed to gaslight you. Community is where we disrupt that.[8]

Polyvagal Theory

I'm sure we can all attest that the pleasures we feel in social relationships of different kinds—parent-child, friend, or lover—are crucial to our happiness. According to the United States Association of Body Psychotherapists, traumatic stress literally rearranges the brain-body connection specifically in areas dedicated to pleasure, trust, and engagement with other people.[9] Socializing is a key aspect of well-being, but danger turns off our social engagement system—basically our ability to enjoy banter, play, and intimate connection with others.

We may be able to channel fight-flight-freeze anxiety into activities such as housecleaning, shoveling the driveway, or working out at the gym, but we're now learning that these activities are even more healing when they involve other people we trust. For all the talk about self-care these days, we need to remember that it doesn't mean we have to do it alone; when we pair self-care activities with people we enjoy, they can be all the more meaningful.

This is explained scientifically by the neuroscientist Stephen Porges's *polyvagal theory*. *Poly* means "many," and *vagal* refers to the vagus nerve. It's been called the "wandering nerve" because it's a long cranial nerve with two branches that provide essential bidirectional information between the body and the brain. The vagus nerve is connected to three different neural circuits—social connection, the ability to mobilize, and the ability to relax. The *dorsal vagal* branch of the vagus nerve goes into the back of the brain stem and into the gut—think survival. The *ventral vagal* branch of the nerve goes to the front of the body and face—think safety after we've been triggered—and it wires to the heart to help us feel bonded with others. It seems bodily safety, a sense of ease, and trusting others are interdependent. This explains why we usually want to be left alone when we're on edge but want to kick it with friends when we're feeling good.

Co-regulation

As babies and children, we learn how to gauge whether we're safe or not by reading cues from caregivers—the sound of their voice, eye contact, facial expressions, and body language. This signals our vagus nerve in one of three directions: mobilize, relax, or connect. This is called *co-regulation*, which is a survival strategy by our nervous system to know the interactive cues to trust someone or not. A soft, soothing tone of voice paired with a smile registers as safe. If these interactions are typically responsive, kind, and reliable with caregivers, we grow up more trusting in our adult relationships. Early experiences may shape the nervous system but ongoing experiences can reshape it. Even the co-regulation with our pets—how we talk with them and make eye contact—can soothe our nervous system.

I've explained how our nervous system listens through different channels of awareness—inside our body to what's happening in our viscera and outside to the world around us. An example of both of these is *neuroception*, the unconscious vibe we pick up between us and another person. An example of this I see often with my clients is when one partner comes home in a good mood but the other comes home grumpy. Next thing you know, they are both crabby and snapping at each other. What happened? They "fed" off each other. This is neuroception, our nervous system and our social system coming together in a subconscious way. You could think of it as our social engagement nervous system.

Fortunately, the more bodyful we are—recognizing these internal and external signs, such as the way someone alarms, confuses, or calms us—the more clever we can be in turning to safer relational experiences. We can ask to be held, rocked, or snuggled by those we trust, or we can create stricter boundaries and avoid people we don't trust. And as I'll explain more in chapter 10, our body's sensory system plays a big role in discerning our pleasure with others, whether it be the visual perception of a face, being touched by grooming, or smelling something wonderfully familiar. These meaningful and safe experiences are what rewire an overactive stress response.

Our Three Brains

In case your mind isn't already blown, I've got more to say about the mind! Or at least the brain, which contains the mind. Neuroscience now suggests we actually have three brains.[10] The one we all refer to at our head is technically called the cephalic brain. Thank it for our thinking, making meaning of things, and creativity. We also have our heart (cardiac) brain, which generates emotions, love, gratitude, empathy, and passion. The heart communicates to the brain in four ways: through nerve impulses, biochemicals, pressure waves, and energetically through electromagnetic field interactions.[11] No wonder matters of the heart can be so all-consuming. And then there's our gut (enteric) brain, which is designed to focus on our sense of self, mobilization, and self-preservation. Think "gut instinct," butterflies in your stomach, or something eating away at you. Your belly ecosystem can regulate your brain chemistry: it's estimated that 90 percent of the body's serotonin (the chemical that brings ease and contentment) is made in the digestive tract and about 80 percent of the immune system lives within it.[12]

Although they play different roles, they're all considered brains because they each have their own nervous system (sensory neurons, motor neurons, ganglia, and neurotransmitters) to take in information, process it, store it, and access it when needed. This explains why some people (myself included) can make quick decisions based on instinct and emotions but then need more time to mentally explain the reasoning behind it.

Integrating all three brains holds the key to decision-making. When you apply them with a regulated nervous system, a consistent movement routine to practice agency, and reliable support, you can reprogram your neural networks and make changes.[13] To have this kind of brain-body influence at your fingertips, accessible twenty-four hours a day, is something we all have potential for. Bodyfulness gives you a systematic approach to synthesize these different voices of wisdom.

The Science of Communal Movement

My client Kareem came to me because he loved tango dancing, which is pretty cool, if you ask me. But the problem was his wife thought it took up too much of his time. Originally, they started doing tango together, but after getting injured she stopped. He couldn't stay away because it was so fulfilling to him—the movement, the blood flow, the energy with someone else, the technical aspects of learning and bilateral use of his brain, the expression of his body. One night, Kareem snuck off to tango class without telling his wife and when she found out, she was furious. Kareem's shame for lying by omission is what led him to therapy. He told me he couldn't bear to give up tango; it enlivened him and took away his stress. I was torn as well. How could I possibly suggest he stop doing something that was a huge source of vitality for him? Turns out, I didn't. But I did help him learn to have better communication with his wife about his needs and ways they could engage in other physical activities together.

The power of dance was clear to Kareem. Whether it be dance, canoeing, or an outdoor concert, the opportunity to practice moving in rhythm with others can lead to interpersonal (syncing with the group) and intrapersonal (matching one's own breath and movement) flow, which are both powerfully pleasurable. Think of the times you swayed with the crowd at a music concert, shimmied alongside someone on a dance floor, sweated with folks in a workout class, or sang a song with people at the piano. Perhaps you *haven't* done those activities, in which case you might want to give them a try; communal moments of song, dance, and flow are enlivening and connect people to the human spirit, a type of collective intimacy.

Once while leading a women's circle, I kicked it off with my Head, Heart, Gut, Groin Moving Meditation (see page 277). Afterward, a woman remarked that it made her migraine fade away. Was it her body's movements, the support of community, or both? Research is confirming the beautiful benefits of movement with others, igniting social connection, expressive freedom, strengthened self-esteem, and togetherness. For example, dance movement therapy has been shown to reduce feelings of depression, and simply moving with others has been shown to help our self-esteem.[14] When people sing together there's a collective resonance that leads the brain to let go of separateness and increase connection. It's remarkable how people's brains synchronize and increase their sense of unity. As the psychiatrist Bessel van der Kolk said, "Americans use alcohol and drugs to treat PTSD. But other cultures turn to dance, song, music, and drumming. And yoga shows greater effectiveness than any pill you can take."[15]

While on the topic of pleasures being enhanced by others, I'll be discussing intimacy, sexual health, and eroticism in the last few chapters. Here I will add that both emotional and physical intimacy thrive when your nervous systems (parasympathetic, sympathetic, and enteric) is in balance, otherwise vulnerability with someone else becomes much harder. Sexual intimacy involves a beautiful oscillation process between your nervous systems that leaves you both relaxed *and* excited in the best possible sense. No wonder it can feel so enlivening.

Even though science is showing us the potency of embracing our primal selves through motion, alone and with others, many disciplines shy away from the healing powers of bodily movement and the experience of pleasure. It seems there is still a fear for our animal selves. To be afraid of that part of us means we're afraid of our own innate healing, vibrancy, and erotic energy. Although many somatic practices caution that vigorous movement could trigger unresolved trauma, it's clear that incorporating dynamic movements, sounds, and social engagement is essential for us all to awaken.

THE SCIENCE OF CHANGE: WHAT FIRES TOGETHER WIRES TOGETHER

Ever wonder why it's so hard to make certain changes? Sure, there is the seduction of comfort and the fear of uncertainty, but it's also because long-held patterns become more deeply ingrained, like the roots of a tree that thicken and spread farther into the ground. Patterns that have been around longer, such as those since childhood, were created by neurochemicals "firing" together repeatedly. There's a saying: *what fires together wires together*. It's called "Hebb's theory," after the neuropsychologist Donald Hebb, who said in 1949 that neurons that ignite or fire at the same time will then partner with each other. Focusing on something causes your brain's reticular activation system to red-flag all things related. Their repetition forms and strengthens behaviors and beliefs, causing us to learn and adapt *or* repeat. The brain figures that if you are repeating something, it must be significant, so it strengthens those connections (like when a new song is played incessantly on the radio and you learn the words). This is why I suggest we fire and wire together the types of pleasure I've discussed to offset our bias toward negativity.

Discernment

People avoid making changes if they think it will take too much effort. We want revolution in three easy steps. As my Grandma JuJu used to say, "Bit by bit the bird builds its nest." But what if you knew you could feel better after a matter of minutes? It doesn't take much movement to ignite a small shift that creates a ripple effect mentally and emotionally.

Crossing the threshold from *diving in* to *discharging* and then *delighting* requires discernment and consistency. Discernment is about nuanced judgment and refined awareness; it grows from practice and learning from our past. The first time I went to an acupuncturist, he took a quick look at my tongue to inform where to put the needles. I asked him how he could glean much of anything with just a glance. He explained, "When you've seen as many tongues as I have, you don't need more than a second." This applies to your bodyful practice. Like a pilot logging hours, the more regularly you listen to your body, the easier it starts to become. Your somatic toolbox gets expanded, and you become more skilled at knowing which tool to grab when something needs attention. Configuring what goes in your toolbox comes from inquiry that asks, "Hmmm...do I need a little of *this* or do I need a little of *that*?" Developing interoceptive awareness and discernment involves asking yourself lots of questions.

Over these last two chapters I've shared how Western medicine is starting to recognize that the body and brain are always in conversation with each other, always alternating from a bottom-up approach starting at the body and a top-down approach starting at the brain. The challenge is how to apply this truth in the real world with real people. As psychology tries to figure out *how* to apply it, the stages of bodyfulness offer a road map. In upcoming decades we'll continue to pull back the curtain on the role of the body to heal emotional issues and expand compassion. My hope is someday it will be probiotics, not Prozac; movement will be our medicine; and our body will no longer be marginalized.

~ 9 ~

Motion Is Lotion

Our bodily genius is a premiere decision-making tool, a
navigation device extraordinaire, an agent of release and
healing, a wisdom carrier of deep insight, and the holder
of secrets and mysteries.
                                                —*Michaela Boehm*

SO FAR WE'VE FOCUSED on our relationship with the physical body,
a place of infinite potential, and what can be cultivated when we truly
listen to it. I've just shared with you some of the Western science
supporting bodyfulness and now we switch gears to the *energy* of the
body, a more reverent, nuanced lens through which ancient cultures
understood what it meant to be wholly and fully human.

The philosophies I'll be sharing here—Ayurvedic medicine and
the chakra system—have inspired bodyfulness with perspectives that
enhance our understanding of the body's language and connection
with others. Ayurveda is one of the oldest holistic healing systems,
dating back at least five thousand years. It recognizes that the elements found in nature are also within you, that the times of day and
the seasons of the year influence everything from the quality of your
sleep to the quality of your sex, and that good digestion is critical for
optimal health (think enteric brain from the last chapter). The chakra
system, composed of seven main energy centers located deep in the
body, describes the different energetic patterns that accumulate in the
body. These energy patterns are the residue of everything you've ever
thought, felt, experienced, or acted upon and they influence the way
you show up in your life (similar to body memory in the last chapter).

These are complex theories, so for our purposes I'll only be sharing the highlights of each—as they pertain to bodyfulness and our ability to embrace pleasure. If they jibe with you, I suggest exploring them in more depth on your own. They've stood the test of time and certainly have something to offer our modern, hectic lifestyle.

AYURVEDIC MEDICINE

Americans spend $3.5 trillion a year on health care, with pretty much every penny spent *after* the problems happen.[1] Seems clear that if we don't take time for our wellness, we will be forced to take time for our illness. What if the US tried to solve problems by looking systematically at the big picture, focusing on the cause, not the symptoms? As a holistic health model, Ayurvedic medicine got this long ago, emphasizing prevention by looking at factors such as diet, sleep schedule, detoxifying movement, lovemaking, and daily rituals. Both Ayurvedic medicine and bodyfulness aim to prevent future wear and tear while also naturally helping with stress recovery.

The word *Ayurveda* means "the knowledge of life," and comes from the Sanskrit words *ayur* (life) and *veda* (science or knowledge). Rather than a "one size fits all" approach to health, an Ayurvedic physician focuses on the *whole* person—body, mind, and spirit—and their connection to their environment. They recommend dietary and lifestyle changes and herbal support, based on any imbalances they perceive. These imbalances come from stress, trauma, poor choices in relationships, and anything that goes against or clouds their elemental nature.

Each one of us is a unique combination of three energetic qualities, or *doshas*, called *vata, pitta,* and *kapha*; each of which is made up of two of the five fundamental elements—space, air, fire, earth, and water. This combination is established at conception and is known as our *constitution*. Vata is made up of air and space; pitta, fire and water; and kapha, water and earth. Everyone and everything have some of each dosha, although generally most people will have one or two that predominate. For example, if you're pitta-vata, then the fiery nature of pitta may be joined by the moving force of vata. This is called your *dosha configuration*, and it's based on your temperament, disposition, physical traits, and emotional style, tempered by the seasons, lifestyle habits, and relationships. Noticing how these elements shift in and out of balance within you over time can guide self-care practices and ignite deeper bodily connection.

Your constitution might be more air (vata) if you are creative, alert, restless, love trying new things; if you graze on snack foods, have a thinner body type, are more easily chilled, have a hard time sweating, have dry skin, and aren't the best sleeper. Your constitution might be more fire (pitta) if you are competitive, ambitious, witty, courageous, focused; if you take the lead, have an athletic build, have soft skin, sweat easily, and run warm. Your constitution might be more earth (kapha) if you have a stable temperament and calm energy; if you are caring, thoughtful, a good leader, and a kind listener; if you have a fuller or heavier body type, have good stamina, love to collect things, and can sleep for long periods of time.

Curious to know which type you are? Take the Ayurvedic Dosha Quiz at the end of the book and see the suggestions based on your results. Combine it with self-inquiry, such as "How is my sleep schedule working for me?" and "How do these particular foods make me feel?"

STOKE YOUR FIRE

I marvel at how Ayurvedic medicine recognized the importance of digestion long ago while modern science has only recently "discovered" how central it is to our psyche. Ayurveda sees a natural diet as key to vitality, especially how well a person assimilates their food. The gut is where your inner fire (*agni*) resides and so naturally you want to keep it stoked and burning bright. Ayurveda recommends ways to do that with the following suggestions:

- Since cold foods and beverages shock your digestion, eat and drink warm things to help your organs of digestion and elimination operate smoothly. (Chinese medicine agrees.)

- Start your morning with half a lemon squeezed into a glass of warm water to gently rev up your digestive process.
- Add spices to your cooking, specifically anti-inflammatory ones such as turmeric, cumin, coriander, fennel seed, and cardamom.
- Regularly eat yogurt (think probiotics) and clarified butter (ghee) to aid the healthy enzymes in your belly.
- Chew your food slowly and thoroughly. It's recommended to take about thirty chews per bite. That's probably about twenty-five more than what most of us frenzied folks do in the US.
- Make lunch your main meal of the day to give you sustained energy and so digestion doesn't interfere with your sleep.
- Pharmaceuticals weren't an option thousands of years ago, so obviously they aren't a part of Ayurvedic medicine. But Ayurveda does believe in *plant medicine* such as ashwagandha to help with fatigue and curcumin (the main ingredient in turmeric) to help with inflammation. Both antioxidants come from roots, but you can buy them in capsule form. And maca powder helps with energy and stamina. It's always a good idea to consult with a holistic doctor before taking new supplements.

RITUALS

No matter your dosha, Ayurveda is a big fan of daily routines to cleanse and calm you, so I suggest you experiment with them to see how they land. Some aspects may not resonate, such as their belief in a vegetarian and pro-dairy diet; it's fine to disregard them. Many suggestions are simply common sense that take little effort. Here are some for all dosha types:

- In the morning, splash cool water over your face to feel refreshed.
- Use a tongue scraper to take off the night's decay and promote oral health.

- Go to bed around 10 p.m. and wake up around 6 a.m., or when the sun rises. (I certainly have trouble with this one.)
- Use a neti pot to cleanse your nostrils and help you breathe more fully through your nose. Not only do the nasal pathways serve as filters to pollutants in the air compared to breathing through your mouth, but nose breathing tells your nervous system you're in a steady, calm state (compared to mouth breathing's message to enter a stress response).
- Self-massage your whole body with a warm, natural oil such as coconut oil or unfiltered sesame oil to remove toxins from your body. (But if you're short on time, you could just do your feet or face.)
- Take baths regularly to soothe your muscles.
- Spend time in nature to calm you and connect with the earth's beauty.
- Move your body every day with stretching to release toxins. (After all, Ayurveda is called "the sister science of yoga.")

THE AYURVEDA-YOGA CONNECTION

I first learned about Ayurvedic medicine during my yoga teacher training. More than just a form of exercise, the sequences in yoga are intended to cleanse the internal organs, prepare people for still meditation, and balance the doshas (as well as the chakras, which I'll share later in the chapter). For example, backbends and warrior poses are heating for air types, forward bends are cooling for fire types, and twists help stimulate stagnation for earth types.

Much like Ayurveda, yoga comes from an ancient five-thousand-year-old philosophy that integrates the mind and body rather than viewing them as separate operating systems. A typical flow yoga class pairs breath with movement, a great way to get blood flowing and discharge stress with moving meditation. It's just as much about mental flexibility as it is about physical flexibility. As you breathe through the poses, you learn to tolerate deep sensations, rewiring reactive patterns. Your focus on the steadiness of the breath alongside your muscular dynamics gives you a break from a chattering mind. There are a ton of yoga styles and yoga teachers out there, so mix and match to find the right one for your body. The physical practice can also be a gateway to apply yogic philosophy, which encourages reflection, nonreactivity, self-compassion, acceptance, service, and surrender. I have found that what traditional exercise, mindfulness, and interoception lack is this philosophy of befriending and engaging the body the way yoga does. Yoga has changed my life for the better in ways I still struggle to put into words.

SEXUAL ENERGY AS VITAL ENERGY

Speaking of movement, Ayurveda encourages a rich sex life—or lovemaking, as they call it so exquisitely. Lovemaking is seen as one of our most primal and essential needs, with the power to nourish us. Rather than a Western attitude around sex of shaming or taboo on one end and salacious and performative on the other, Ayurveda sees sex as a sacred form of expression and a valuable physiological release to give us *ojas*, vital energy and immunity. Sexual expression helps us expand to a higher level of consciousness. If any of our channels are blocked (such as poor blood flow or constipation), sexual energy is dampened.

Ayurveda also believes we absorb the other person's energy through physical intimacy. It's common knowledge that people's moods can rub off on us, so why not believe that sexual energy can be transmuted to the other person? This belief is shared with the philosophy of tantra, also a five-thousand-year-old Hindu practice, focused on the weaving and expansion of energy that occurs with intimacy. One branch of tantra pertains to tantric sex, which contrary to popular misconception is not just the art of erotic love but the merging of sexuality and spirituality. Orgasm is not the point—unlike our modern, goal-oriented lovemaking, which sees orgasm as the whole point. But when it does happen, it's more than just a physical release but a way to imbue your whole body with vitality.

I was so intrigued about this idea of energy being transmuted during sex that I spoke with Katie Silcox, an Ayurvedic expert and author. She explained that Ayurveda believes sex is both a partnership and an unconscious psychological agreement to exchange sacred energies (called *cords*) and information between people. This really gives new meaning to the phrase "cut the cord."

Silcox elaborated that Ayurveda and tantra view sex as a particularly sacred choice for women. As life givers, women's biology makes them especially sensitive to the giving and receiving of nourishing energy. If a woman feels lovingly tuned in to her partner, her body will release *amrita*, her natural lubrication, beautifully translated as "holy bliss nectar" (and "flower moon water" in Taoism). The synergy a woman has with her partner impacts not only her amrita but also her ojas, which is important for her maternal health. Her womb and fluids are like a sexual gatekeeper; no amrita, no sex. Women's comfort matters.

Whether this idea reveres women or complicates their sexual freedom even more is debatable. Either way, it never hurts to consciously pause before engaging in any kind of partnership with someone, including a romp with a new flame. Listen to your body, whether it be your intuition or your fluids, to inform sexual decisions—not in a punitive, proscriptive, shaming sort of way, but as an invitation to explore your inner voice regarding who you're drawn to, when you want to be with them, and why. It's an opportunity to connect with your body's wisdom—what you notice before (your sexual cravings or hesitation), during (your physiological response and amrita), and after (your energy and ojas).

DOSHA COMPATIBILITY

Ayurveda believes that sexual desire and needs differ from dosha to dosha, and that the amount of sex you have depends on the time of day and season. (Perhaps my dosha quiz at the end of the book should be standard screening material on dating apps?) Afternoon is better than morning or evening because it doesn't interfere with optimal energy and sleep. I tend to agree; most people aren't in the mood at the end of a long day or a filling dinner. Ayurveda also believes winter and spring are the best seasons to have more sex because it builds energy, heat, and ojas, something you already have more of in the summer and early fall.[2] You just might save money on heating bills that way.

Air types are considered more sensual and free-loving, with a wavering libido. They get by with the least amount of sex. Since they can get bored in the bedroom, air types need to mix things up by having more spontaneity and adventure. For them, the sillier and more surprising the sex, the better. But they tend to be more depleted from orgasm and prone to dryness. They can also take more time to commit to a relationship. But once they do, they're all in.

Fire types have high libidos and tend to be passionate, but they can burn themselves out. They're more visually stimulated, so setting makes a real difference for them. Because of their driven nature, it's important they balance out their red-hot lovemaking with some calming activities that tap into their sensuality and slow them down, such as massage and meditation (otherwise their ojas get depleted).

Earth types tend to have a lower libido, which can take a while to get revved up. One teacher said that they're like freight trains—it takes a while to get them moving but once they do they're unstoppable. They can have sex every day with their stamina. Kaphas tend to be nurturing, sensual, and romantic, geared for long-term relationships, but they are more likely to get attached too easily.[3] More than the others, earth types feel better sexually when they have a vigorous exercise routine and avoid rich foods. For all types, if you're not in the mood, it's an invitation to check for imbalances, not a time to force things.

Beyond lovemaking, relationship dynamics can be improved when you understand the different doshas. People might find their pitta partner too overwhelming, kapha partner too loyal, and vata partner too capricious. Take a vata-kapha relationship: for the vata person, it's in their nature to be chatty and restless. Meanwhile the kaphic person—naturally quiet, steady, and stable—wonders why their vata partner can't just slow down and take a breather, and feels frustrated they aren't a better listener. In turn, the vata partner wishes their kaphic partner would initiate things and be more excitable.

Knowing your partner's dosha can help cultivate empathy and appreciation for them rather than blame and resentment. You can see their behaviors as part of their elemental nature, not simply their "fault." If your life experience hasn't taught you this already, let me be the first to say *you can't change your partner*, at least not core aspects of them. So rather than attempting to, try to see your differences as complementary. Knowing the ways people are influenced by their dosha, in and out of the bedroom, can be handy as you find, or maintain, a pleasurable relationship.

CHAKRAS

A central idea in the history of psychology comes from Abraham Maslow, a psychologist who suggested in 1943 that humans have a hierarchy of needs. He said we are all motivated by five basic categories in the following order: physiology, safety, love, esteem, and self-actualization (living up to our human potential). It's long been visualized as a pyramid, with food, water, warmth, rest, security, and protection at the bottom; then belonging, friends, and lovers; and at the top is respect and being your best self. I like to picture it as a mountain: your base provides strong support, while your summit encourages upward life direction. If your basic needs are satisfied, you're free to focus on things related to meaning, purpose, community, spirituality. . . and life's pleasures, of course.

Pleasure is the ultimate renewable energy.
—*Gayatri Beegan*

The chakra system operates on a similar hierarchy, believing there are building blocks to nourish higher aspects of our well-being, but it operates in the *subtle energetic body*. For some folks, it feels off-putting to conceive of energy or a "subtle" body they can't see or touch. Our culture has a lot of skepticism toward anything we can't prove scientifically. I'm not talking about the words of a Magic 8 Ball or the movement of a Ouija board but the ability to sense energy inside you and in the space around you. Ever felt someone looking at you even though you couldn't see them? Ever got a strong hit of romantic chemistry? Things you can't see in a tangible way but you know when you feel them? It's actually part of our evolutionary survival to have this instinctual awareness. Once you cultivate energy awareness, it can become a helpful guide.

This idea of energy can be interpreted in different ways, but the gist is that we are more than just our physical form. We are all rhythmic beings; and everything in nature, including humans, vibrate at different frequencies. As Albert Einstein said, "Everything in life is vibration." And as I said in chapter 6, our body is an ecosystem linked together through nutrient cycles and energy flows. I'm not talking about energy in terms of metaphysics or mysticism but rather the oscillation in our body at all times to keep things functioning optimally.

Pause now and see if you feel the oscillation of energy inside of you. One way to start is by listening to your heartbeat, your pulse, and the nerve endings on your fingers as you hold this book.

You can also think of energy in terms of your mood. All of our emotions are different types of energy. They give us valuable information, and once we realize that they're seeking recognition—the very thing we're not all that enthused to do—they can start to pass. So, like a crying baby soothed by rocking and cooing, give them compassion. Once, I began a client session with a meditation and she began to tear up right after I said the words "subtle body." She later shared that my simply mentioning this deeper part of her gave it permission to release.

ENERGETIC BOUNDARIES

Relationships are certainly sources of energy, whether it be the charge of attraction, the tingling of romantic chemistry, or the way someone's presence calms us. I think of screen time as the opposite of relational energy. It's tiring for many reasons, such as eye strain, focusing on one spot, not moving for long periods of time, and being alone (typically). It's draining because it lacks the vitalizing power that comes from a human-to-human experience. Relationships are physical, biological, and chemical, just like us. They are a gathering, a hug, a place to come together. You can't bottle this or summarize it in a text. This energy—not computer energy—is what boosts our sense of meaning. The challenge is to keep connecting to our bodily energy and synergy with others in this era of rugged individualism and technology.

Understanding your energetic language helps you have body boundaries between yourself and the outside world. The word *boundaries* gets tossed around a lot, but it's ultimately about anything you have a right to and a responsibility for (such as a right to your body and saying no to touch). The circumstances guiding your yes or no (your limits) can always change but what you're responsible for does not change (your body, thoughts, feelings, etc.). The more bodyful you are, the more you know what your boundaries and limits are because your body will tell you when they've been crossed. For example, if someone enters the room with a warm smile, your jaw and belly might soften as you smile back and feel more present, signaling you can have a more open body boundary. Someone else might come along and interrupt you as they try to sell you something in a pushy way. In this case, your throat might get dry and your stomach might tighten, signaling you to keep your distance (creating a body boundary). I see this as related to neuroception, which I described in the last chapter.

Boundaries are crucial to self-care, relationships, and resilience. Take empathy as an example: you can feel so much empathy for the suffering of the world that you become depressed and depleted. Energetic awareness within the lens of bodyfulness encourages your self-preservation; it helps you notice how much you have to give before you run out of reserves and hit rock bottom.

THE SEVEN CHAKRAS

Now that I've made my case for energy, here's the nitty-gritty on the chakra system to get you going. According to the Sanskrit scholar Christopher Wallis, our modern understanding of the subtle body and the chakras grew out of tantric yoga, which flourished between

600 and 1300 c.e. Over time, Westerners have put our own spin (so to speak) on these spinning wheels of energy.

Chakras (Sanskrit for "wheel" or "disk") are spinning within you at all times. From a Western viewpoint, this corresponds to where nerves collect and where electrical activity is high. There are seven main chakras starting from the base of the spine and moving up to the crown of the head. They influence one another, similar to Maslow's hierarchy. You can also compare this to the energy system of Chinese medicine, which believes we all have channels (meridians) of energy, or qi (pronounced "chee"). And like the fluid nature of the doshas, the energy in each of the chakras can become excessive or blocked. There can also be patterns among them, such as blocked energy in the first three chakras at the lower part of the body and excessive energy in the chakras at the upper part of the body, which is a common pattern I see among overthinking, sedentary professionals.

Our bodies are in constant flux between balance and imbalance. Noticing an imbalance in one area will help bring the others back into balance. Since everything within us is oscillating, if there is a blockage, energy flows are restricted. Think of something as mundane as your vacuum: if the suction tube becomes jammed with too much lint, it gets clogged in one area and doesn't work well. The same can be said for energy blockage in your body. Energy becomes stagnant if you ignore the body by being too sedentary or stuck in your head, or excessive if you're too impulsive and don't invite some rationality.

These bundles of nerves at each of the seven chakras reflect our psychological, emotional, and spiritual states in that moment. Occasionally I do chakra readings in my office with clients using a pendant over their seven chakras, watching for patterns in movement. Sometimes this isn't necessary because their life circumstances make clear where their energy imbalances are. I had a client whose cousin tragically died from choking. Soon after, my client developed constant sore throats, tightness in her upper chest, and a hacking cough. Her heart and throat chakras were affected. In addition to processing what this sad loss meant to her, we also engaged in chakra-balancing exercises that honored the way her grief manifested as physical ailments, in order to help her cope more fully.

Other examples of chakra patterns include: frequent constipation, which may indicate a blocked first chakra; and frequent headaches, which may mean your sixth chakra is blocked. An incessant talker who has a hard time listening may have an excessive throat chakra. Granted, these manifestations could also be symptoms of a junk-food diet, dehydration, or being drunk, respectively. This is why understanding your own energy patterns is just *one* of the many elements that help you develop embodied mindfulness and releasing/balancing methods. The more you're able to see all the factors in life that influence you, the better your ability to discern what you need moment by moment, a hallmark of building the interoception necessary to be bodyful.

Since I can't emerge from this book like a magician and give you a chakra reading, check out my descriptions and suggested practices in the appendix to help balance your chakras.

~

I once heard the yoga therapist Bo Forbes say that we live in an *epidemic of disembodiment.* She's not talking about being decapitated, of course, but about the ways we perpetually detach from the layers within our body. This can especially be the case for our deeper energetic layer. The somatic psychologist Alexander Lowen understood this when he said, "Without awareness of bodily feeling and attitude, a person becomes split into a disembodied spirit and a disenchanted body." For most of us going through the motions of life, we are far from enchanted with our body or embodying our spirit.

There is this beautiful and mysterious reality within the resonance of your subtle body. What if you embrace what unfolds there rather than ignore or control it? As twentieth-century philosopher Søren Kierkegaard so eloquently put it, "Life is a mystery to be lived, not a problem to be solved." These ancient teachings encourage you to explore how to make body connection and movement *all your own.* The suggestions here are like that of a teaching assistant; your body's response is the real teacher.

PART THREE

~

Soulful
Reconnection

~ 10 ~

Leave Your Mind and Come to Your Senses

Memories establish the past. Senses perceive
the present. Imaginations shape the future.
—*Toba Beta*

WHILE PERUSING OPTIONS in a brochure for a writing center, I came across this description for a creative writing class that enticed me: "Heat. Abundance. Excess. Juice. Long hot nights, cool rivers, the moon the only witness. Feel adventurous and sly . . . take an excursion into the belly of your life." Why, yes, yes, I want to do that! Those twenty-seven words didn't exactly make logical sense, but they evoked something sensual within me, which kicked my imagination into gear.

Our senses simmer below the surface. In this case, merely imagining a sensual experience transported my body and mind to the exotic. Connecting with our senses leads us down a variety of paths, some eliciting pleasure, some evoking pain, and some causing disgust (as in the case of Charlie the dog from chapter 2). Given that humans are wired to avoid pain and seek pleasure, and given that life presents us with both, it's common to find ourselves on a seesaw—chasing yummy sensory stimuli on one end and avoiding yucky sensory stimuli on the other. Not to mention that sensory enjoyment is also context—and person—dependent. For example, tickling (stimulating the sense of touch) can feel silly and playful in one context or painful and aggressive in another. Or when I was a kid, both. I would beg my dad to turn into "Tickle Monster." It was pure belly laughs until it suddenly wasn't and I was begging for mercy. Our senses have strong opinions and make sure we know it.

STOP TIME TRAVELING

An old parable describes a man traveling across a field who encountered a tiger. He fled, the tiger after him. Coming to a precipice, he caught hold of the root of a wild vine and swung himself over the edge. The tiger sniffed at him from above. Trembling, the man looked down to where, far below, another tiger was waiting to eat him. Only the vine sustained him. Then he saw a luscious strawberry nearby. Grasping the vine with one hand, he plucked the strawberry with the other. Oh, how sweet it tasted.

Most of the time, we take our senses for granted, completely forgetting we're sensate beings. After all, who has time to stop and smell the roses? As a busybody myself, I've gone through phases in which I couldn't be bothered to slow down and sense my way through the day, let alone register I just wolfed down lunch. When we're striving to accomplish too many things, our head is basically time-traveling to the next task and the next one . . . Aside from trauma, as I described in chapter 7, there are a couple common things that kill sensuality: (1) being in a hurry, and (2) being on autopilot. Both are examples of the time-traveling mind—meaning you're dwelling about the past or projecting into the future so much that you've robbed yourself from being in the reality of your life. (I chuckle to think of how one of my clients went to her psychiatrist for a medication refill and referenced her time-traveling mind, given we'd been working on it together, and her shrink literally thought she was referencing a psychotic episode.)

Being on autopilot most often happens when you're in familiar settings such as taking the same driving route to work or going through your bedtime routine. It's a form of checking out—you're in your car or brushing your teeth, but since you don't need to consciously remember to turn left on Fifth Street or put toothpaste on the toothbrush, you end up daydreaming about random people, places, and things. You're zoning out thinking about a work email or why the kids aren't asleep yet; you're certainly not pausing to feel the toothpaste glide along the smoothness of your teeth. You're just as unaware of your senses when you're in a hurry. Rather than being in the moment, you're all about getting to that next seemingly important thing, such as the emails waiting in your inbox or showing up on time for your doctor's appointment. In both of these examples of a time-traveling mind, you've become pretty detached from your body and are wandering through your thoughts. Given all you've learned about pleasure and bodyfulness, you can see how your mental chatter cuts you off from the language and wisdom of your body and from presence overall. Slowing down and being bodyful by noticing each of your senses helps you (1) feel tuned in to the moment, (2) manage sensory input you don't like, and (3) welcome more sensory input you do like.

Voluptuary: One whose life is devoted to sensual appetites; a sensualist, a pleasure seeker.

SENSUALITY: TO EACH THEIR OWN

But first I'll share with you part of my journey to understand the wide world of the senses. I went through a phase where I turned gatherings with friends into opportunities to sneak in a little field research. Let me say, in my defense, I'm pretty much "off the clock" when I'm socializing. I am *not* analyzing you—at least not any more than the average person might. Granted, I sometimes ask probing questions, which can make people squirm a bit, but that's also just part of my curious personality. Typically these gatherings were women, or a mix of men and women. Sometimes the guests were in partnered relationships, sometimes not. Sometimes people arrived single but left with a prospective mate by the end of the night, thanks to the matchmaker in me. Every type of relationship status or lack thereof was fair game for my research.

On a night that included men and women from jobs ranging from producer to dentist to professor, I waited until the wine was flowing and the conversation felt more spirited. Then I explained that I was doing some exploring about sensuality and asked if they would mind sharing with me what has been their *most sensual moment*.

The question was first met with blank stares; no one seemed to want to be the first to respond. If there was a thought bubble over their heads it might read, "Is she asking me to tell a *sex* story?" I wasn't entirely surprised. We live in a culture that typically equates sensuality with sexuality, and requesting them to tell a sexual anti-dote would have been a bit intimate for this mix of acquaintances. So I explained that sensual does not necessarily mean sexual, although it can include their sexiest of moments if they choose, such as an erotic moment alone or with someone else. I reminded them that a sensual moment is really anything related to each of their senses, like the smell of the ocean or the texture of their dog's fur. It's any experience where they felt heightened awareness of one or all of their senses and that led them to feel awake or alive. For some, the hesitation was about the fact that it had been so long since they had felt sensual. I mean, really, the manic pace of life in the US doesn't exactly encourage being leisurely and sultry.

Even though being sensual is not the same thing as being sexual, it's still personal and requires some vulnerability to talk about. After all, I asked a question about a topic people don't usually share with others; a topic about a moment that touched their heart. Every time one person shared their story, it encouraged others to do the same. So as they dug into the crevices of their memory, we heard nostalgic stories on themes including:

Dipping into a rushing river
Kissing a lover
Star gazing
Childbirth
A wilderness cabin
Carving turns while snowboarding
Hiking a mountain
Lighting candles
A stormy night

Collective grief at a memorial

Hands in clay

Singing in the shower

A sudden moment of clarity after a difficult decision

When it's quiet and I notice feeling present

The thrill of trying something new

Taking ecstasy with my girlfriend

Petting animals

Ocean waves on my feet

Submerging myself underwater

Read back through the list again. Which ones evoke something in you? Can you describe that "something"? If so, is there a place in your body where you feel it, such as a change in your breath or a release in a tight muscle?

This list represents a wide array of moments from the simple and solitary to the exotic and erotic. It illustrates the endless possibilities that exist when you stop to notice, and later recall, those moments of being in your aliveness. How? Being sensual connects you to your natural self in the present moment instead of that time-traveling mind with the story lines. Although, yes, there is mental time-traveling involved here in order to remember, you're experiencing it physically in the moment rather than creating it in your mind based on the need to control, plan, or prevent things in the future because of past threat or regrets.

Your senses are connected to the real-time primal self inside your body. These visceral messengers make emotional "sense" of your life experiences by connecting to your immediate surroundings and then producing a response within you, a sense perception. This creates a feedback loop between your brain, mind, and your body.

Sensual presence is about listening to your body's needs. They let you know when you need to lean into emotions and pleasurable sensations and when you need to lean out to protect yourself.

Similar to how mindfulness is about listening to your thoughts free from judgment, try listening to your sensations simply as they are to see what they're telling you. Are those wool socks too scratchy? Is the guacamole not spicy enough? Does hearing that song fill you with nostalgia? This should sound familiar: stage one of bodyfulness entails listening. Understanding these bodily cues helps you self-regulate. Stage two of bodyfulness entails balancing through types of release or containment.

Being connected to your senses fine-tunes what kind of response is best in the moment, among all the options and exercises you've been learning. For example, yoga movements extend your field of perception by stimulating nerve endings and sensory perception. Your repertoire of movements might change with the seasons and day of the week. With practice you'll learn how each of your activities stabilizes or enhances your senses in a different way, supporting you overall. For example, one of my clients was working through her fear of flying. Sense by sense we made an action plan for her to calm herself during her flight. She wore clothing with textures that soothed her, made a calming playlist, packed some snacks that felt like comfort food, brought essential oils that helped settle her, and got an aisle seat so she could frequently get up and stretch. This is using your senses to your advantage.

You're probably too in your head right now, in fact. Take a breather and tap into what you see, hear, taste, and touch. And then notice what you feel in the moment overall.

After reading the list of my guests' most sensual experiences, you might be thinking, "Cool, but life can't *always* be like a perfume commercial." Valid point. Life is *not* always Charlize Theron floating on a cloud in a billowy gown as she promotes perfume. Nor is it always a pharmaceutical advertisement—the Viagra commercial where the man gets a hole in one on the golf course, then dines with his lover (foreshadowing his next hole in one).

There are moments when you'd rather not welcome your sensory experiences—not one iota. These range from being agitated by horns honking in the street to flinching when someone startles you from behind to being caught in a sudden downpour. It seems it's more the exception than the rule to ignore our senses or to be suddenly reminded of them when something irritating happens. Which is why I liked doing this exercise with my guests—it gave them the opportunity to dig into their sensual memory in a *fun* way. Given that our brains cling to the negative and shimmy off the positive, we all need to remember the delicious moments more often.

Where it becomes tricky is when you feel discomfort or pain. The last thing you want to do is welcome or stay with those sensory experiences. With pain, most people disconnect from their body in a whole slew of ways. As I mentioned in chapter 7, in psychotherapy lingo we call this *dissociating*, which means escaping, numbing, or avoiding in a trancelike state. It's your couch-potato self, zoned out watching TV while snacking, paying little or no attention to what you're eating, how it tastes, or your level of fullness. When in pain, people will shut down from their senses and become frozen or reactive. Some may get worn down from too much sensory stimulation. For example, highly empathic or intuitive people are ultra-tapped into sensory perception, including other people's vibes, and this can be exhausting (which is why boundaries are key).

We all have times when we're provoked by our senses, which ranges from annoyance—for the person who hasn't suffered a major trauma—to intense fear—for those who have. This was the case for my client Cindy, who had been working with me individually for several months. At one point, she decided the time was right to have her husband join the sessions since he wanted more physical intimacy. She had experienced repeated sexual abuse as a small child and this radically shaped her sense of safety. So much so that she didn't have any. The world was just not safe. There was an invisible line drawn around her, and if anyone got too close or touched her, it was incredibly provoking. Her rigid body was like a barricade to the outside world. Understandably, this did not foster intimacy with her husband. By the time Cindy brought him to our session together, they'd been married for seven years and, to my surprise, had a child. She explained that conceiving their son was one of the few times they'd ever been sexually intimate. The three of us met, and at the end of our session I *thought* I was moving slowly by asking him to gently rest his hand on hers. After all, their goal was to have more physical touch in their relationship. Cindy's reaction to his hand indicated otherwise.

What would be a seemingly kind form of touch was a cause for alarm for her. Cindy's nervous system reacted as if she was that four-year-old being violated once again. How would her nervous system know any different that day in my office, given she'd shielded herself from touch for so long? It never had opportunities to experience similar scenarios that were safe and pleasant, and it had no way to change the associations to help repair the damage. Your body responds to familiarity—good or bad—and picks up where it left off, unless you've done body-based trauma therapy to dislodge the past and rewire your response.

The next time you feel afraid or set off because a new experience is bringing up unresolved emotions, notice your reaction. Is your immediate response to freeze or shut down? To run away from your sensations and feelings? Given that your body's natural response to stress is to fight, flee, or freeze—and freezing doesn't allow you to complete the stress cycle—it's important to engage the second part of bodyfulness, discharge. Think of the phrase *fluid, not flooded.* You want to release the stress from your body through any number of movements, sounds, or breathing, to move that stress through you until you're able to remove yourself from the triggering sense(s). Whether the movements are fast or slow is up to you and what you need. (Refer to the "Fluid, Not Flooded Exercise" in the appendix for examples.) This completes the stress cycle and teaches your body you are better capable of handling stress. So, the next time you're bombarded by sensory stimulation, try to stay fluid, have some type of discharge plan, and seek co-regulation from pets and people you trust to help give you containment.

For some people, the issue is less about managing their senses than it is about avoiding feeling them in the first place. Ask yourself, "What prevents me from noticing my sensations?" Busyness . . . past stress . . . being overwhelmed . . . guilt . . . not wanting to be bothered? If this describes your experience, here are some suggestions to sense your senses:

Take your tongue and rub it along the smoothness of
    your teeth.
Close your eyes for the first two or three bites of food.
Look at the textures, colors, and shapes immediately
    around you.
Wash your hands slowly or splash your face with cool water.
Massage your scalp.
Look up at the sky, day or night, and notice what you see—
    the clouds, a sunset, the moon, or the stars.
Look at the horizon, especially after staring at your screen
    for long bouts of time.
Notice what's touching the bottom of your feet. Give each
    foot a mini massage.

PRATYAHARA

In the yogic tradition, *pratyahara* means "sense withdrawal," which is not about cutting yourself off from each of your senses but about learning to go inward, withdrawing from all the commotion in the outside world. It's different from creative fantasy or dissociating. It's about noticing your sensory experience but not reacting to it, labeling it, or engaging with it. I sometimes explain to my clients that it's the difference between starring in the movie as the action hero and watching the movie at a distance, from the safety and comfort of your seat. You're the observer to your self, versus being the reactor. Set the intention to *respond instead of react*, which is a life practice. Can I get an amen?

One way to explore pratyahara that's getting more attention lately is a flotation tank, also known as a sensory deprivation tank. It's a dark, soundproof tank, filled with a foot or less of salty water, that you lie in for anywhere from sixty to ninety minutes. Benefits include reductions in stress, depression, anxiety, and pain and increases in optimism, mindfulness, and sleep quality.[1]

I decided to give it a try. First, let me admit I'm not a fan of confined spaces, which I discovered the first time I tried a sweat lodge in Tulum, Mexico. After about ten minutes in that cramped, pitch-black teepee, I ended up trampling over people between me and the doorway because I couldn't get out of there fast enough. A few years later at the Esalen Institute, the conditions were different and I'm proud to say I was able to stick it out. I had heard good things about the flotation tank, so I decided to do some research of my own. If I can do it, I'm pretty sure you can too.

I showered, got naked, and entered what looked like a cross between a coffin and that large space-shuttle egg that Robin William's character Mork from *Mork and Mindy* arrived in. The water was a nice warm temperature. I was ready to surrender myself to the ninety minutes that lay ahead.

It took a while, but over time I noticed that something within me kept intercepting my mental babbling. My mind would wander and then my breath would interrupt it, each time releasing my inner tension a little more—so essentially the opposite of my default dynamic. I felt somewhat naked and exposed—oh wait, I was!—not in a scary way but in a way that let me surrender and release emotions I had been avoiding. These were emotions I kept below the surface—they had been peeking out here and there, but I wasn't giving them much attention, because quite frankly they were challenging. But in the floatation tank there was no holding back. And that was okay. It was simply okay. No additional story line. I accepted the emotions and the circumstances they came from, and that was that.

Turns out what I was experiencing was akin to what Zen monks experience when they meditate. My brain was going into theta waves, which are "patterns of oscillations generated by the combined electrical energy our neurons produce constantly."[2] This is why I was able to simply allow everything to surface that needed to, with no need to control it or hold back. The type of brain wave you're in represents a different physical and mental state.

At the same time, I felt a deep sense of gratitude that rather than distracting from my emotional challenges, I was meeting them. I was feeling them. I was "doing the work," because I understood that avoiding it no longer benefited me. Like most people I know, when I'm feeling peachy, or even status quo, I'm not motivated to do the inner work. But when I'm confronted and realize there is no false refuge to hide in, that's when I hunker down and—Do. The. Work. As I floated, my gratitude swiftly turned into a type of raw beauty of the healing process I was experiencing and the healing process in general that's available to all of us. I had been cut off from remembering the tenderness that comes from getting through the emotional work to the other side because I was hiding behind the logistics of life. Yes, therapists do this too.

A couple years later, I tried the floatation tank again, during a time of life transition and heartache. It was a very different experience, but again a tender one. This time, as I lay weightless in salt water, my hands naturally floated themselves to my heart center, one on top of the other, as though they wanted to contain the literal ache within that sensory membrane. As if there wasn't enough salt in the tub, tears streamed out of me. The release made my body even more buoyant. I thought of the book—and later, the Daniel Day-Lewis movie—*The Unbearable Lightness of Being*. Within the heaviness in my heart, and the things that had been weighing me down, I embodied a little lightness here in my Mork and Mindy space-shuttle egg.

Science may not know exactly what a floatation tank does for us, but I believe there's something to be said for stripping away all the noise, sitting (or floating) in your silence, and letting what needs to flow through, flow through. I know firsthand that although I left that night with my same life transitions and sad heart, I felt better. Emotionally I was in a place of sleepy surrender, and physically I felt a softening in my chest and muscles that only a much-needed release could provide.

SOUND

I told my friend Micah he was a bit of a music snob. He responded matter-of-factly, "I don't judge people who like different music from me. I judge people who simply don't like music." I got his point. Some part of us is closed off within if we close ourselves off to music overall, given how primal it is. And while the love of music is universally human, it's also deeply personal. Certain types of sounds vibrate melodiously with some people and grate discordantly with others.

What I've observed—in myself and my clients—is that the more open someone's heart is and the more they're connected to their senses and their feelings, the more they let music in and let it touch them. On the days when music falls on deaf ears, I'm typically closed off or buckling down. It's as if life has already demanded too much from me so I'm stuck in my head (even though the very thing I need is to blow off some steam with a dance or a song). For some, playing music when deeply sad or stuck is helpful. They play some melodies and feel better. Music has sensual associations that transport our brain waves and mood.

On some of my past retreats, I've had each participant tell me one of their favorite songs at the beginning of the week. Then I instruct them to play that song at some point during the retreat while by themselves and notice how their body wants to move or sing along. On the last night, we'll have a dance party by a bonfire on the beach and I'll share a playlist I made of their songs. Everyone gets an opportunity to hear their favorite song played and share it with others. People who are tired, perk up. People who don't even know the other person's song, sway or hum along. When it's their song, they take ownership of it and do their thang. Granted, it helps that we've just finished a week of connecting to our bodies. Some people had already started venturing out of their comfort zone and making friends with others in the group. These are all ingredients to help even the shyest person feel a little braver—perhaps for the first time ever—to dance and sing with a group of people.

Try this for yourself at home. Pick one of your favorite songs, one that matches your mood, and let yourself flow and sway or bounce and twerk—whatever your body is asking—without a damn care for what it looks like. Feel the vibrations. Bonus points for singing along to the words, at least the chorus, which you probably know if it's one of your faves. The sound you make helps you release any visceral stuck energy in your throat—that bottleneck between your head and your heart. This might help prime you to make guttural sounds, such as sighing or humming, when you need that release later during a more hard-to-tolerate moment. These are all ways to help you practice expressing yourself overall, including asking for what you want and need from other people.

I agree with my friend Micah; it doesn't matter what you like musically, it only matters that you let music into your heart from time to time. According to a 2011 article published in *Nature Neuroscience*, when you listen to music, your brain releases dopamine, the brain chemical linked to reward and motivation. Even the anticipation of listening to music causes a release of dopamine.[3]

Sound shows up in our lives in all sorts of ways besides music of course, and one of those ways is the sound of someone's voice. If someone's talking agitates you, consider whether you're focusing on what they're saying or how they say it. *Prosody* is the science of speech expression, including intonation, tone, stress, loudness, pitch, and rhythm. Research has shown that someone's voice can have a real visceral impact to the listener.[4] I once had a client who was easily triggered by her boyfriend's voice, particularly when he was overly excited or annoyed; his voice dis-regulated her. Over time, she was able to regulate herself by pausing and practicing bodily release, and her boyfriend became more aware of his tone putting her on high alert. On the flip side, someone with a monotone voice can also send cues to a person's nervous system that they're not safe because of the *lack* of inflection. Awareness of the role of prosody can make a big difference in communication dynamics.

TOUCH

Most yoga teachers know the power of hands-on adjustments to their students. When I've touched students to help deepen their experience in a pose, they typically melt. Often the release is especially strong at the end of class as they give themselves permission to let go. I don't touch people often, and some I don't touch at all because they've indicated they don't want to be touched. For others, I might sense it could activate their trauma history, or they're new and I haven't had the opportunity to gain their trust. Conversely, when I'm wearing my psychologist hat, I don't touch people at all due to the code of conduct for that profession. Ironically, this rule shows just how much the licensing board recognizes the power of touch, for better or for worse.

Touch reveals our deepest attachment wounds. Professionals know that babies and children who lack touch are damaged throughout their lifetime, because touch reduces stress hormones (cortisol) and blood pressure, calms the nervous system, and increases contentment and resiliency.[5] Going too long without touch—called *touch starvation* or *affection deprivation*—as an adult is also harmful to your health.[6] In the right moment, touch creates human bonds and helps us feel cared for. Sometimes when people crave and chase after sexual touch what their soul actually yearns for is simple and loving forms of healing touch. Something to remember when sex is not an option, or at least not a nourishing one.

Among all the senses, touch reminds us of our body boundaries most strongly. When it's welcomed, it can feel like nurturance (a hug) or therapy (a massage). When it's not, it can feel like a violation. Kind touch soothes and supports, but it can also trigger older pain, like it did for my client Cindy when her husband touched her hand. This gives literal meaning to the expression "He rubs me the wrong way."

Not all touch is created equal and neuroscience confirms it. Skin is the largest organ in the body, full of receptors that sense touch. It's connected to the somatosensory system, part of the sensory nervous system. David Linden, the author of *Touch: The Science of Hand, Heart, and Mind*, explains, "There are two touch systems, one that gives the 'facts'—the location, movement, and strength of a touch—and we call that discriminative touch."[7] For example, Cindy registered her experience as light touch, on top of her hand, and that it didn't move.

There's also this really cool emotional touch system. It has special sensors called *C-tactile fibers* that give information more slowly. It's vague—in terms of where the touch is happening—but it sends information to the insula, which is like a mail sorter classifying types of touch to our social bonding system. Different sets of sensors and nerve fibers register with different parts of the brain to determine it was a "hug from a friend," versus "cheeks squeezed from your mother." According to the neuroscientist A.D. Craig, it's this area of the insula where "people sense love and hate, gratitude and resentment, self-confidence and embarrassment, trust and distrust, empathy and contempt, approval and disdain, pride and humiliation, truthfulness and deception, atonement and guilt."[8] A bad taste or smell is sensed in the frontal insula as disgust. A sensual touch from your beloved is transformed in the back of the insula as comfort. The insula is also the part of the brain that helps you connect with music; people with lesions to this area don't resonate with music unfortunately.[9] In which case my insula must be blessedly lesion free.

Not only does the *type* of touch make a difference but where the touch is happening influences whether it feels like a feather or a firecracker. The part of your brain that processes touch has a map of your entire body surface, but it's distorted. Linden explains, "It over-represents areas that have lots of fine touch receptors (like the face, the lips, the tongue, and the fingers) and under-represents areas that don't have many receptors (like the small of your back, your chest, and your thighs)."[10] This helps explain why we have highly pleasurable "erogenous zones" in our body, which we'll discuss in the next chapter.

Touch is probably the most gendered of the senses. For example, most men have been socialized to believe that sexual touch is the only acceptable (i.e., masculine) form of emotional expression for their body. Other types of touch, such as hugging or holding hands, were considered too feminine. This is too bad, because it prevents males from having a way to connect with their feelings and then give and receive physical comfort in ways other than sex. So they're cut off from their feelings and the power of touch to soothe them or their partner. How truly limiting and sad when men and women alike are confined to some human expressions and not others. Loving touch is essential in ways most people don't have the words for.

Apparently our touch receptors peak around age eighteen and then we lose them slowly as we age, so don't delay getting as much touch as possible! Whether you have a partner or not, you can snuggle in the texture of your bedding, give yourself a neck or foot massage, and exfoliate your skin. If touch is overstimulating for you, keep going back to the sequence of somatic steps in the "Fluid, Not Flooded Exercise" in the appendix for people who need to calm their sensory system.

SIGHT

Although we walk through life looking around, how much are we actually seeing? Unless you're tripping on mushrooms, you might not be fascinated by the colors popping or the juxtaposition of an image against another. Even as a culture that emphasizes visual first impressions when it comes to mate attraction, we've now become so lazy we take merely seconds (or less!) to decide if we want to swipe left or right.

Your eyes are a portal to your brain about what's happening around you and this contributes to what later becomes your memories (with a bit of reconstruction mixed in). But did you know that purposely looking at something soothing is also a way to distract from your anxiety? In the sensory exercises I listed earlier, notice that a few of them include looking at the sky or objects around you, as a way to give you a fresh perspective and ground you in the present moment. Interestingly, having *too many* visual distractions won't help you: a recent study suggests that distraction can change our perception of what's real, making us believe we saw something different from what we actually saw.[11] What your eyes see sends your system information about your environment, but how you look to others gives them pertinent information about you. Eye contact is a communication all its own, whether it be come-hither eyes, a penetrating gaze, or an eye roll. The eyes really can be a window to your soul.

One of the best ways to connect to your other senses is to *close* your eyes. Notice how your awareness of taste or touch is heightened when you do, because you're able to hone your focus.

TASTE

If you lost your ability to taste, what would you miss the most? This happened to a friend of mine and it wasn't long before she stopped having cravings or caring about food. She was just eating to live (not nearly as enjoyable as living to eat). Our sense of taste is connected to survival. We're primed to spit out something that tastes nasty as a way to prevent getting sick. Food can also be a work of art—as anyone who's enjoyed a spicy Indian curry or tried to perfect a French coq au vin will tell you.

Eating food can certainly be a sensual act. I watch my mom, who has dementia, as she's being fed. Lacking the ability to form coherent sentences, she communicates her pleasures and limits for how much she wants through her facial expressions and pace. She often closes her eyes, taking small bites and chewing very slowly. Her days as a working parent eating on the go are over; she has nowhere else to be, and it's likely the highlight of her day, so she takes her sweet time.

We could compare our sense of taste with food to our sexual behavior: sometimes we eat more sensually and slowly, sometimes we devour it ravenously to quickly meet our needs. Sometimes we need more variety, a little spice to get our juices flowing. Cooking together is like foreplay—the finished product displayed like someone revealing themselves in new lingerie. We also notice our taste receptors when we kiss someone. *Besos!*

Americans rarely eat together anymore. In fact, the average American eats one in every five meals in their car. Eat more often with others, taking your time, and enjoy the experience of savoring it together. It nourishes your body and heart.

SMELL

Smell is the sense most associated with memory. This is because our olfactory system is located in the same part of the brain that affects emotions, memory, and creativity. According to the Sense of Smell Institute, smell in the form of aromas, fragrances, and scents can promote relaxation, reduce stress, improve alertness, energize, relieve pain and depression, reduce inflammation, and kill disease-causing microbes.

They identified the top twenty smells that make people feel happier. A few of these might make you hungry: freshly baked bread, clean sheets, freshly mown grass, fresh flowers, freshly ground coffee, fresh air after rainfall (seems something being fresh is significant), vanilla, chocolate, fish-and-chips, bacon frying, roast dinner, babies, lemon zest, lavender, apple and blackberry crumble in the oven, a freshly lit match, roses, party poppers and—the weirdest two of all—rubber tires and petrol.

Within smells there are pheromones—"nature's perfume." Many species use smell and scent to detect when their mate is ovulating as a sign of "sexual readiness." Apes and dogs will smell the behinds of their mates, while giraffes will smell a mate's urine. In humans, a study found that men who smelled shirts worn by women ovulating (which produced something called *copuline*) had higher levels of testosterone compared to men who smelled shirts worn by women who weren't ovulating.[12] So, to the ovulating bodies out there, depending on what you want to attract the next time you head out, you might want to think more about your decision to wear perfume or go au naturel.

INTUITION

On my initial client paperwork—right there with their sleep habits, medications, intentions, and everything else—is a question on whether they trust their intuition. I want to know because if they don't, it's important for us to work on cultivating such a valuable skill. Why? Although there's debate about the neuropsychology of our intuition, it's believed to come from the *ventromedial prefrontal cortex*, a region that stores information about past rewards and punishments. So if we're connected to intuition, it means we're listening to the signals in our body based on the past and are able to make better choices moving forward.

Often referred to as our "sixth sense," intuition is that initial pre-thinking sweet spot within us. It's a visceral inner knowing before the analyzing mind steps in with bias. Intuition exists in the absence of outside "proof," confirmation, or persuasion from someone else— it's all our own. After all, you are the expert of you. *Intuition* comes from the Latin word *intuir*, which means "knowledge from within." Intuition has been described as a "distinctly human and highly complex, poorly understood" ability.[13] I believe Albert Einstein said it best when he proclaimed, "The intuitive mind is a sacred gift and the rational mind is a faithful servant. We have created a society that honors the servant and has forgotten the gift." There's noticing it, listening to it, then acting upon it. This voice inside your heart and your gut says that you know what to do. It's a matter of having the courage to follow through with what it says.

~

It's hard to fully open your channels of sensation in a world that's constantly bombarding you with discord of different kinds. Perhaps the best approach is how the novelist James Baldwin describes it: "To be sensual, I think, is to respect and rejoice in the force of life, of life itself, and to be present in all that one does, from the effort of loving to the breaking of bread."[14] You may not be able to control all the construction sounds and kids crying, but you can find moments to create your own sanctuary. Available to anyone at any time, our senses are a catalyst to awaken our body on a deeper level.

~ 11 ~

Give It to Me, Give It to Me: The Desire Chapter

Possibility is where desire lives.
—*Saida Desilets*

SIMILAR TO MARRIAGE VOWS, what if you created vows for your relationship with yourself? Think about what inspires you and tickles your fancy. Also notice habits that have helped you feel your best in the past—whether it be a certain amount of sleep, staying hydrated, meditating, or whatever. Pick a few that have had the biggest impact and consider these your *nonnegotiables*. Then reflect on a few things that have been essential to you in relationships—respect, humor, kindness, etc.—and make them your relationship nonnegotiables. Be creative and have fun with these; unlike legal vows you'd have to say in front of your Aunt Betty Lou and Uncle Bob, these are aspirations, not rigid rules. Light a candle, throw on an outfit that makes you feel sensational, write them on nice paper, and toast yourself with some bubbly. (I'm always looking for more ways to incorporate effervescence.)

You could also envision yourself on a dreamy honeymoon to bask in the glory of your personal promises. Maybe you never had the fantasy honeymoon you always dreamed of, but that doesn't mean you can't give it to yourself now. That's what I did; I gave myself a do-over for my honeymoon, which had been more like a honeygloom. The trip ended in Bali with my husband telling me he lacked any romantic feelings for me. Even though we were now finally done with his medical residency, he couldn't resuscitate our spark.

So, as cliché as it sounds, I created my own *Eat, Pray, Love* experience. I went back to Bali, seven years after my honeygloom, for a yoga retreat with my favorite teachers. This time around I enjoyed Bali for all the magic it had to offer, undistracted by a disengaged hubbie. I had the perfect blend of time to myself with movement, music, delicious food, and new friends. It gave me the chance to reflect on just how much I'd grown and learned since Bali visit number one. My business had flourished, I had developed a spiritual practice, and I had learned more about my relationship patterns (a lifelong practice for us all). I once heard the poet David Whyte suggest that to your soul, it doesn't matter if you succeeded or failed, it only matters that you lived life your way. I've thought about this statement many times, and it always gives me chills. It certainly wasn't an easy path between my first and second visit to Bali, but my soul felt more content.

Your soul is the epicenter and collective voice of your senses, desires, appetites, affections, and character. You can't *think* your way to soulfulness; you need to slow down and intuit your soul's voice as your truth and invite it as a guide. Review your unchanging essence from the first section of the book to start connecting more to your soul.

Here you are at a place in the book that has led you to see more clearly what your soul wants—for inner connection and intimate connection with someone else. On the surface level, we all want to feel good. On the soul level, we want to feel deep connection, love, and desire, mutually. But as you've read, there are all sorts of reasons we don't have the kind of intimacy our soul craves. So, the first step is to connect to what *you* desire in the first place, right? Not quite yet.

I MATTER . . . THEREFORE I DESERVE

The first step is acknowledging that you *deserve* to desire, because you are a righteous human, worthy of wanting and receiving in the first place. As a therapist, I've witnessed just how often people don't feel deserving, sadly. Our original definition of the word *deserve* might have something to do with why that is. The word originated in the thirteenth century from English and Latin (*deservire*) with *de* meaning "to devote oneself" and *servire* meaning "to serve." The definition implies you have to do something to warrant receiving, like self-sacrificing and doing things for others—which we definitely need on a collective, global level—as long as it's done in balance. Otherwise giving away too much of yourself leads to burnout. Receiving self-care and support from others is rejuvenating and prevents you from getting depleted. It's a wise person who's in touch with their own internal needs and drives. I say it's time we *servire* ourselves just as much as we *servire* others!

This is key because healthy relationships are not one-directional, they are not about only serving the other person. (That would be a master-slave situation and not in the "kink" sense.) It's about understanding how healthy and vital it is to give and receive. That back-and-forth energy creates something dynamic and flowing. In this mutual effort you create intimacy. If you struggle to receive compliments, gifts, or other good fortune, you're interfering with how that person (or even the universe) wants to honor and connect with you. And you probably don't have an accurate sense of yourself.

Some people operate with backward reasoning, believing that because they haven't had a soulful lover (at least not a satisfying one), they must not deserve one. In the absence of answers and linear circumstances, our brains fill in the blanks with all sorts of skewed reasoning, often blaming ourselves, others, or the world in general. You wouldn't find it logical to believe you didn't deserve sunshine just because you're in a rainy season, so why believe you don't deserve your desires for intimacy because you're lonely?

There are people who may feel deserving of love, but they struggle to validate their desires or to receive what they crave erotically without guilt. For example, Brandon came to therapy because he felt disconnected from his body and from pleasure during sex. He was in a healthy committed relationship with Gretchen and didn't want to blow it because he was sheepish sexually. In our first meeting he shared two factors that explained a lot: he was raised Catholic, and he grew up in a small Midwestern town. Catholicism taught him most people are sinners and should feel ashamed of themselves. (On the upside, as Billy Joel sang in his song, *Only the Good Die Young*, sinners are at least typically more fun.) He had learned lots of good/bad and right/wrong thinking. That religious doctrine, combined with his geographic influence—a mix of Scandinavian and German—encouraged stoicism, modesty, keeping his head down, and not asking for much.

No wonder when I posed the question, "What do *you* want?" he was flustered. This was certainly not the first time I've seen that question throw people off. People look at me like I'm an alien. Turns out the verb *want* is quite loaded. Seems *what do you want* are four powerful words.

For Brandon to focus on what he wanted—beyond day-to-day survival needs—felt indulgent to him. Even his motivation to come to therapy was to please his partner, not to figure out and own what *he* wanted. I asked him if he felt that he *mattered*, and he said yes, but it was a recent acceptance. For Brandon, him mattering was not the same as deserving something as "luxurious" as pleasure.

One of my favorite mantras is SO HUM. It translates to "I matter." Inhale as you say to yourself the syllable SO and exhale the syllable HUM.

There are a few key questions I frequently ask in sessions to get at the root of things. Such as this one: "What would it mean if you were someone who . . . [*was vulnerable . . . was angry . . . said no . . .* etc.]?" In the example of feeling deserving, notice if you associate it with being entitled or greedy. For Brandon, it meant he was selfish. Being chaste and self-sacrificing is what makes you a "good" person. Remember those messages from the anti-pleasure preacher in chapter 3? Willpower and abstaining equals good. Craving and being permissive equals bad. Brandon felt he already had so many opportunities and privileges in his life, that to feel he deserved more—in this case, mutually pleasurable intimacy with his partner—would mean he was asking for too much.

Having a hard time identifying and asking for what you want can stem from feeling that you're already *too much*—too needy, too demanding, too unsatisfied with what you have, too emotional, taking up too much space, and so on. This may have begun if you had parents who wanted you to be seen and not heard, so you buried yourself. Or because parents or a past partner implied you were too much, probably because they couldn't (or wouldn't) meet your needs. Or because your religious upbringing—Catholicism, in Brandon's case—equated wanting more with being bad, wrong, greedy. So with the onset of sex, when Brandon's body would instinctively want to express its desire, he would override it by leaving his body and overanalyzing in his mind.

This leads to another key question I often ask clients, especially for people who "check out" during uncomfortable moments: "Where do you go when . . . [*you aren't in your body during sex, you're bingeing on food, your partner is sharing their feelings* . . .]?" Brandon and I realized he would leave his embodied experience and become an evaluator of his performance, judging what he was doing and *especially* judging what he wanted. So he blocked himself from acknowledging it by going into his worried, criticizing thoughts. How unpleasurable.

We discovered Brandon had a fear that if he let himself succumb to pleasure it would mean his willpower for other important duties could go down the drain and lead to a path of no return. Even though he didn't think of himself as someone with an addictive personality, there was still apprehension. Brandon's fearful belief isn't unusual. I often see clients go from one end of the spectrum to the other when trying to change a behavior. For example, someone who's never let themselves show anger might overcorrect and suddenly have angry outbursts. So cut yourself some slack. If you've been told your whole life that you could *never* have sweets and then suddenly in the dining hall at university you're staring down a table full of desserts to choose from, you're probably going to go hog wild. After a while, you get tired of stomachaches and cavities and the desserts are no longer such a novelty anymore (I might be speaking from personal experience here). Whether it be desserts or desires, it takes time to eventually trust yourself and your ability to strike a balance.

On the flip side, there are folks whose biggest fear is that they're *not enough*. They're driven to be more and more extraordinary, stemming from perfectionism. (I always say, "perfectionism is for robots, not humans.") They're so attached to being special (sometimes to the point of being egotistical), that the worst insult you could hurl at them is to imply they're boring. Not only do they want to *be* more but some of them constantly want to *experience* more from life—chasing after excitement and adventure. These tend to be people who know what they want, express it, and feel they deserve it. The problem is they can get over reliant on seeking external validation instead of it emanating from within. For some, the problem is they judge what they receive from others as never good enough (projecting onto others their own fear of being not-enough). Both tendencies ("I'm not enough" and "I'm too much") stem from the same core wound that who they are, as they are, is not okay.

WORTHY

For both camps, not only are you enough but you are *ultimately* enough, of you, in the best possible sense of the idea. The experience of desire—recognizing it and asking for it—is so inseparable from the experience of self-worth. It means recognizing your "light," the things you like about yourself. Then integrating that with your "dark" (sometimes referred to as your "shadow"), the things about yourself you find hard to accept. If you can integrate the two because you know it's *all part of being human,* then you won't be stuck in shame for having a shadow to begin with. We all have one, because we're always expanding and evolving through life. With Brandon, and with other clients I've worked with on self-worth, I help them accept their humanness, meaning that all humans are in a constant state of learning and growing from their mistakes, and that we're all working toward our potential.

Think of self-worth as a healthy sense of entitlement to everything from basic human needs to more pleasurable needs. "I deserve to take a break right now after working all morning," "I deserve to go on a walk to stretch my body"—these are not grandiose needs. Recognizing this and tending to your needs is the foundation for letting yourself enjoy pleasure for the sake of pleasure. Recall the chapter on play when I talked about the importance of non-outcome-/non-goal-focused behaviors to boost creativity and playfulness. That applies here. Identifying your desires and experiencing pleasure from them is not about producing, measuring, or creating results for others, just as being playful isn't necessarily about someone else's needs. Your own moment-by-moment satisfaction exists and matters for your sake (and obviously you need to be sure there's not undue harm to others in the process). These moments are not a waste of time. Remember, each one aids in your long-term resiliency and overall sense of joy.

For example, I recently went to a Korean spa to try their "V Steam." Yes, the *V* stands for *vagina*. You velcro yourself into a gorgeous cape that covers you from the bosom down, sit on a large throne-like chair with a hole in the middle of the seat, and receive a warm steam with essential oils that releases for a half hour. I called my friend on the way home and she laughed, implying it was all a sham. I tried to convince her otherwise, explaining that it touts healthy hormone production, protects the uterus from ulcers and tumors, helps with irregular cycles and hemorrhoids. Then it dawned on me: Why do I even need to convince anyone else of my enjoyment? Why would I need to justify my desires for some fun novelty? The whole production, including the meditative room it was in and the hot tub afterward, was worth it to me. The Buddhist author and teacher Pema Chödrön suggests the key to an engaged life is to remain curious—and so I was. So what if the V Steam didn't supercharge my pussy; it satiated my curious desire to experience it and my whole body felt refreshed afterward.

DESIRE AND BODY MEMORY

As we discussed earlier, your body keeps the score. Your blocks to worth, desire, and pursuing pleasure typically relate to blocks in your body. In Brandon's case, his fear of giving in to pleasure was also bound up in his body memory. When he was three years old, he was diagnosed with leukemia. For a couple years the poor little guy had to go through all sorts of intrusive treatments to fight the illness. How confusing and disorienting for a child. He distinctly remembers getting spinal taps. His dad would hold him down during these painful procedures. From a nervous system perspective, his body went into freeze mode. Being held down prevented his body from its natural inclination while stuck in a trauma: engage in fight or flight to return to safety. For that whole time—between three and four years old—his mind and body came to equate deep sensation with pain. So as an adult, his body associated *all* types of deep sensation with pain, including the kinds that come from pleasure. While physically intimate with Gretchen, he would reactively compartmentalize. It was his four-year-old self stepping in to protect him.

I encouraged Brandon to do yoga classes more regularly alongside our work. This helped him practice remaining in his body when he felt deep sensations. For example, while he was in more challenging poses such as Chair or Plank, he would focus on staying in them longer each time, taking deeper breaths to ride the wave of his sensations (recall the idea of titration I mentioned in chapter 6). This was all part of the process to help him feel more empowered in his body and trust that he was in charge—he got to decide whether he wanted to take a rest or not. He was no longer stuck like his three-year-old self had been. Brandon was rewiring the connection between physical sensation and pain and overriding the automatic reaction of leaving his body and engaging his mind where he could safely get lost in thoughts. Alongside this, he did complementary therapies such as myofascial massage to release bound-up connective tissue where the trauma had been lodged.

As for his communication with Gretchen, we worked on Brandon expressing his opinions with her about day-to-day matters such as what to eat for dinner or which route to drive. Over time, this translated into him feeling more comfortable voicing his desires in the bedroom. While she had always loved his sensitive nature, Gretchen craved a little more alpha energy in the bedroom. She started digging his newfound masculine energy. Eventually they were more in tune with each other and this was reflected in their erotic life.

DEFINING SEXUALITY

At this fourth type of pleasure, which is also about the third stage of bodyfulness, connecting to desire, pleasure, and sexuality can feel like a foreign language for so many of us. Many older folks probably haven't thought much about their sexuality other than to identify as straight or gay. So let's start from the very beginning.

Everyone has some sort of relationship with sexuality—good, bad, neutral, or "it's complicated." The word *sexuality* encompasses sexual orientation, gender identity, behaviors, preferences, desires, eroticism, libido, physiology, social narratives, cultural and religious/spiritual beliefs, clothing, fantasies, and surely some other things I've left out. Your sexuality can evolve too: fluid or fixed, something natural or innate, or something learned from outside influences (as we discussed in part one). Often someone's sexual preference can be constant, but their libido can go through peaks and valleys, so don't put a lifelong label on yourself or someone else as promiscuous or prude.

I'm not a big fan of labels in general, but sometimes having a descriptive name helps you better understand a concept. Here are some terms, outside of traditional ones such as *heterosexual* and *homosexual*, that describe sexual preferences:

- *Omnisexual*: Diverse in what turns you on. It could be people, places, or things. All bets are off.
- *Demisexual*: You don't experience sexual attraction unless you feel emotionally connected. The term comes from being "halfway between" sexual and asexual.

- *Pansexual*: Attracted to people regardless of their gender or being nonbinary. It comes from the Greek word *pan*, meaning "all."
- *Sapiosexual*: Sexually attracted to a person's intellect or mind before appearance.
- *Hetereoflexible*: People who are primarily into the opposite sex but are open-minded and it depends on the context.
- *Asexual*: A lack of sexual attraction for people. They can still have romantic attractions and enjoy sex with someone even while not being attracted to people. Asexuals still experience physical sexual urges independent of another person. An "aromantic" asexual is not physically *or* romantically drawn to anyone. This is different from celibacy, which is a decision to refrain from sex.

These are descriptors, but no one should feel stuck in one category or the other. You can call yourself pizzasexual for all I care (a food worthy of desire, in my opinion). These terms are about helping you channel your desires in a world of options. What's most important is that you acknowledge and accept where you're at without judgment, because there's really nothing to judge.

WHAT DO I WANT?

Once you accept that you are indeed deserving, you're now in a much better place to ask, "What do I even want?" If you've been tending to others' needs for so long, you probably haven't thought about it much. Noticing and giving yourself what you want doesn't mean you're selfish nor does it mean you should feel guilty. You've done nothing wrong. Self-care and self-desire activities fill up your tank. Once filled, you're ready to rev up your engine and go places that can help others as well.

Let me help you turn on the ignition. For years I had a column in a couple newspapers titled Ask Dr. Rachel, which focused on wellness and relationships. Here are just a few common things people asked me about desire:

- How do we maintain the initial exhilarating phase of dating for as long as possible (the butterflies, the blushing, the giggles)?
- How do I get started pleasuring myself?
- I have a lively fantasy world. My partner does not. How can I help him be more open to experimentation and talking about sexual fantasy?
- What if I'm not attracted to my partner anymore?
- Fresh in a new scene, off four years from dating. How do I get out of my head, let go, and loosen up sexually?

There's a whole spectrum of things people desire erotically (we'll focus on emotional needs in the next chapter). This list didn't even include more unique fetishes—from being turned on by nursing from their wife's breasts while she's lactating to getting off on forcing someone to eat too much and gain weight. Some desires are not surprising; the number one word googled when people search for porn is *young*, while the least googled word is *old*.

For many people, what turns them on is *being* the turn on. We like to be desired! It's flattering and validating. One of the top fantasies for women between ages twenty and forty is to be dominated and ravaged.[1] Now, obviously women don't want to be violated, but this does shed light on how much they want to be chosen, and by someone with masculine energy who takes charge (just like Brandon's gal, Gretchen). Although the heteronormative style had always been most accepted (male and female having penetrative sex in missionary position), people are naturally interested in variety. In fact, "vanilla" sex (the traditional kind) is now becoming the minority, according to records of searches online. We can credit (or blame) online porn for raising the bar (or should we say, lowering it) by orchestrating the most outlandish, wildest sexual scenes possible for entertainment value. The bottom line is that whatever you like, let your bodyfulness practice creatively connect you to your desires. You do you. Practice with activities that have nothing or little to do with eroticism; if your desire is to eat ice cream in your bed wearing pajamas and not share it with anyone else in the family, own that too.

To help you get acquainted with how desire and eroticism feel in your body, here are some visceral descriptors to prompt you:

Electric charge
Inner fireworks
Flutter in the heart
Awakening
Coming alive
Radiating
Tingling
Fiery flame
Filled up
Ticklish
Feisty
Craving
Magnetic

Did this list conjure up any sensations or visualizations? Feel free to jot down any other words or phrases I left out. Now read this list again, and this time notice where you feel it in your body.

Erotic connection with someone else relies on connecting to your own desires as you experience them—in your body. Sadly, many of us are way too critical of our bodies. If you're shut down and don't want to live in your body, if you think touching yourself is gross, why would you want to invite someone else to join you? Loathing your body sends the message that there's no room at the inn.

Now that you're starting to learn and practice bodyfulness, hopefully you see your body as more château than shack. Hopefully you don't see it as a dilapidated fixer-upper, a problem to be tolerated, outwitted, and avoided, but instead a place of integrity and love, a dwelling of sensation and delight. Maybe, just maybe, you're able to inhabit your body with playfulness and curiosity, like a toy! This is what boys have done with their genitals pretty much their whole lives starting in infancy. Unfortunately, women's genitals being on "the inside" makes the area seem much more mysterious and misunderstood to them. In fact, it's estimated that 90 percent of a woman's clitoris is under the surface and looks like a wishbone. Who knew?! Combine this with the double standards around sexuality for men and women and it often takes much more time for females to feel enchanted with their body sexually.

My first time going to prom highlights just how different teenage boys feel about sexuality in their bodies than teenage girls. At dinner before prom, I noticed my boyfriend would randomly howl like a wolf under his breath to his buddy across the table. Then his buddy would respond with hissing sounds like a snake back to him. My girlfriend and I rolled our eyes, figuring they were just being goofy. We later heard that their shenanigans were because they'd each bought penis puppets, one a wolf and the other a snake. I could never imagine us as seventeen-year-old girls having vulva puppets that we could brazenly joke about. I'm not saying these puppets were inherently bad (in fact, I now think they sound like a fantastic idea to create playfulness for all types of body parts) but that most people socialized as female don't come into their sexually until they are much older and have done some work to get there.

LEFT TO OUR OWN DEVICES

The ultimate way to connect your desires with what feels good inside of you is by practicing self-pleasuring. I have seen over time that masturbation—whether you're male, female, or nonbinary—is a topic where you're damned if you do, damned if you don't. Some clients and friends who have been masturbating since they were young feel such shame about it; some who *never* masturbated until adulthood, or *ever*, feel shame around that as well. No matter how you slice it (or touch it), there are shaming messages about the when, where, and how of sex—and this is particularly true when we're "left to our own devices." Know that it is a natural and healthy part of being human, and there is no right or wrong way to pleasure yourself.

You learned in the last chapter that being in each of your senses, and having a sensual lifestyle overall, connects you to your body and opens you up to the world literally at your fingertips. In this chapter I've shared with you how to explore what you want and deserve erotically. So now you might be thinking, "Alright, Coach, put me in the game." But if the idea of masturbation is something that keeps you on the sidelines, I'm here to walk you through it.

For starters, masturbation is a common behavior. Research from Indiana University found that 40.8 percent of women sampled had masturbated in the past month, while 21.8 percent reported never masturbating before. In another study, only 38 percent of women said they'd masturbated in the past year, whereas 61 percent of men had.[2] Take this with a grain of salt; many studies of sexual behavior struggle to ensure that people are telling the truth, so the statistics could be even higher.

Not only is masturbation common and natural but you're more likely to enjoy physical intimacy with a partner and communicate what you're into if you've already spent time exploring yourself. Another benefit, and this may go without saying, is that masturbation is the safest form of sex because there's no risk of infections or pregnancy. Whatever your relationship status, this type of pleasure has a deserving spot in your self-care routine. Here are some tips to get after it:

- To get in the mood to self-pleasure, consider your environment. You want to give yourself the most optimal conditions. Is the door unlocked? Will the dog be barking to go outside? Is your mother-in-law likely to drop by? Hopefully the answer to all of those is no. Within the emerging world of psychedelic medicine is the concept of "set and setting," which could also apply to masturbation. *Set* is short for "mindset," meaning you want to be in a good place to dive into that psychedelic vortex. If you're raw with grief or have repressed wounds that need to come to the surface, then it's not the best time to trip *or* pleasure yourself. Whereas *setting* is about ensuring your environment is conducive to feeling safe, secure, and distraction-free.

- Create a space of relaxation and calm. Perhaps change the lighting, put on music, and wear something that makes you feel like the hottie that you are.
- Listen to or read an erotic story to boost your libido.
- Use a mirror to check out what's happening at your "wonder down under."
- Whether you're using your hands or a toy, everything's better with lube. Just as I mentioned earlier that *motion is lotion* for our muscle tissues and joints, lubrication prevents irritation or tearing.
- Penetration is often pleasurable for many folks, but about 80 percent of women who masturbate focus on the clitoris rather than vaginal penetration.[9] This is because the inside of the vagina has few nerves at the surface, whereas the glans of the clitoris has eight thousand!
- Try a toy if you haven't already—a wand, vibrator, or dildo are among the most common. Sex toys have always existed to allow people, particularly women, to take control of their pleasure, regardless of whether they have a partner. They give you myriad ways to explore what feels good by adjusting the pace, motion, and size of the toy. There are all sorts of intriguing toys out there. But do your research first because once you take it home and open it, there are (understandably) no givebacks.

EROGENOUS ZONES

We all know our genitals are a direct route to pleasure and orgasm, but remember that there are other ways to achieve this type of pleasure. Particularly for female bodies, enjoyable sex often means focusing on pleasuring the whole body, not just one area such as their genitals. Hyperfocusing on anatomy leaves out all the other erogenous zones. The word erogenous comes from the Greek *eros* which means love, and the English *genous*, meaning producing. An erogenous zone is an area of the body that has heightened sensitivity, which can lead to anything from relaxation to arousal when stimulated.

When people talk about erogenous zones, they usually focus on the obvious body parts, such as the breasts, nipples, clitoris, G-spot, and penis, since these are the sexual areas of our bodies and are more erogenous than others—due mainly to the amount of nerve endings located there. This is because the genitals undergo a process called *vasocongestion*, in which blood flow is increased to these areas, making them highly sensitive when aroused and touched. But there are many areas on our bodies with fewer nerve endings that can still be erogenous and elicit pleasure, depending on the way they're touched, such as the eyelids, forearms, abdomen, and head. Spending time exploring your own body (and your partner's) is a pleasurable way to discover what does or doesn't feel good.

ORGASM: THE GAME CHANGER

Whether it be masturbation or hooking up with someone else, sex is not merely a behavior but a place you go *within yourself*. Nicole Daedone, the founder of OneTaste, which focuses on the art of the female orgasm, said, "We've come to believe that our sexuality depends upon the right external circumstances—a partner who wants to have sex with us, or a body we're willing to let see the light of day. But in reality, sexuality arises from the inside out."[4] This is in line with the first stage of bodyfulness: inhabiting your body by staying present to the messages it's giving you. This is so essential to erotic pleasure you should write it on your bedroom ceiling!

One of the greatest predictors of not only pleasure but also having an orgasm is your ability to stay present in your body. Practicing body presence and giving yourself permission to follow through with what your body wants and needs in other areas of your life will definitely enhance your sexual experience. This sets you up for experimenting with your body and noticing how it responds to different stimulation (types of stroking, pace, different sizes of penetration, more than one erogenous zone at a time being touched, different positions, and different angles . . .). If you have a regular bodyfulness practice (including still and moving meditations) and a regular practice of tuning out a lifetime of sex-negative messages, you're on the road to pleasure town.

Research shows orgasms can increase immune response, help you sleep, quell your anxiety, and heighten your creativity. Talk about the innate healing capacity of the body! When you have an orgasm, your brain releases the hormone oxytocin into your bloodstream, which lowers your main stress hormone, cortisol. So after you have one, stress levels are lower and you're feeling more serene. With less cortisol pumping, your body can do its job of fighting illness and being present. You burn calories, stay limber, sweat out toxins, lower your blood pressure, strengthen your pelvic floor and abdominal muscles, and increase blood flow to the brain. The endorphins released during orgasm act as a natural sedative and diminish your perception of pain. Orgasms also release serotonin and norepinephrine, which helps your body cycle through REM and deep non-REM sleeping cycles. These are the cycles that help fight infection and inflammation, not to mention they make you feel nice and rested. Orgasms are quite a bodily game changer.

Just like erogenous zones, most people don't realize that sexual pleasure and orgasm can come from more parts of your body than you might think. Clitoral, vaginal (or a combination of the two), penile, cervical, anal (for men), and nipple are among the most common. But did you know some people can imagine their way to orgasm without physical stimulation? Even listening to music can induce orgasms! That's called a *frisson*, which is a musically induced effect associated with a pleasant tingling feeling.[5]

Some special attention needs to be given to female orgasms, since research shows it's much harder for women to experience them compared to males. About half of women *sometimes* have orgasms during intercourse, about 20 percent rarely have orgasms during intercourse, and about 5 percent never ever have them. And the other twenty-five percent? My guess is they're probably too embarrassed to participate in a sex study to begin with. In part one I discussed many reasons why this is, from historical, cultural, and gender perspectives. A study from the National Institutes of Health bears this out: "The improvements in gender equality and sexual education since the 1970s have not helped women to become more orgasmic. Neither has the major increase in masturbation habits (among women in general). . . . One challenge for future studies is to understand why women value their partner's orgasms more than their own"[6] Who knows how many generations it will take for this inequality to shift but, oh, how I want to change that.

And how do we explain the difference in the frequency and type of orgasm among women during intercourse? For example, why does direct stimulation of the clitoris more often lead to orgasm than vaginal or combined stimulation? Apparently whether a woman experiences one type of orgasm or the other during penetration could be a reflection of her anatomy, not necessarily her emotional comfort or health. Possibly, the shorter the distance between the clitoris and the vagina (specifically the distance between the urinary opening and clitoris), the more likely a woman is able to have vaginal types of orgasms (G-spot, cervical) and clitoral.[7] This might explain why some women have an easier time experiencing different types of genital orgasms (such as vaginal, clitoral, and cervical) while others are more limited to having only clitoral orgasms.

Position also plays a role—a high percentage of women only achieve a vaginal orgasm while on top, because it's stimulating more friction at their clitoris as well. Another major factor is the way a woman is moving her body. Research has found that a woman's body movement (back and forth swinging movement of the pelvis and chest) is a major contributor to having a vaginal orgasm from intercourse compared to when a woman's body remains still.[8] Once again proving one of my favorite sayings: movement is medicine!

If someone is in better health and has good blood flow throughout their body, they'll be more likely to have genital orgasms of all kinds. Hormonal and genetic factors also have an impact on sexual pleasure. It's quite a multifaceted recipe.

All that being said, I've heard sex therapists joke that they are probably among the least concerned about whether orgasms even happen, at least for some couples. We've seen the problems that result from putting too much emphasis on them. I once had a couple come to me for therapy because neither of them could have an orgasm with the other. They felt emotional intimacy, had great communication, and were attracted to each other, so they didn't understand why they couldn't just have a damn orgasm together. They were especially puzzled because they could typically orgasm by themselves with masturbation. I saw how obsessed they were with "achieving" orgasms together and how they took for granted all the other positive aspects of their relationship. So to take the pressure off, I bluntly told them, "You're giving a lot of pomp and circumstance to something that is technically a muscle spasm." Yes, scientifically, that is what's happening—orgasms happen physiologically when there's continual stimulation that leads to two responses: increased blood flow and swelling (vasocongestion) and the flexing and contracting of the muscles (myotonia). This knocked the orgasm off its pedestal a bit. It turns out the problem was they met in Alcoholics Anonymous. Each of them was so used to having drunk sex—with their inhibitions down because of their "liquid courage"—their body didn't know how to let go during sober sex. Our work wasn't about improving their relationship dynamics so much as retraining their bodies and minds to associate sobriety with unbridled expression of desire.

CLIENT EXAMPLE: SARA

Sara, a straight woman in her late twenties, came to me because she wanted to recover from feelings of shame regarding past sexual behavior. After a long-term relationship ended in her midtwenties, she had a bit of a "sexplosion." She shot out of the gates from her committed relationship and engaged in sex with a handful of different men. These weren't one-night stands—they were more along the lines of short-term relationships with no strings attached. In each encounter she had sex willingly and consensually. By the time Sara came to me, with distance and perspective on her side, she realized what she wanted all along from most of them, more than sex, was attention and to be told she was pretty. Sara's drive for validation led to some fun sexual trysts, but not the deeper emotional connection and self-approval she wanted.

When we explored her self-worth and ability to voice her honest opinion, given how connected the two are, Sara realized she didn't think that saying no in the bedroom was even an option. When people feel disempowered, they lack voice. In Sara's case, men had power over her physically, systemically, and emotionally in her need for their validation. If someone feels another person has power over them, the courage and voice to say "No," "Stop," or "I want something different" becomes blocked. It means confronting the fear of rejection, the fear of getting physically hurt, and/or the notion that it's not okay to say no.

Many women have been raised to believe that saying no and asserting their body boundaries is not an acceptable option. Sonya Renee Taylor's book title *The Body Is Not an Apology* came to her after a friend disclosed that she didn't feel able to say no to unprotected sex and became pregnant as a result. When we don't advocate for ourselves physically and verbally and listen to our boundaries, the consequences can be severe and long lasting. And if women don't feel that they have a right to say no, then they probably struggle to ask for and say yes to what they *do* want. We need a sexual ethic that focuses on being honest and authentic in a relationship as a way to take ownership of our body and its pleasures. The third stage of bodyfulness is about self-confidence, trusting yourself, and owning what you do or don't desire. I'll share more about how to communicate your pleasures with partners in the next chapter.

In our work together, Sara explained that her mom had always been critical of her, which led to an inner drive to be perfect and never feeling like enough. So she spent all sorts of time and money—on her hair, nails, clothes, and makeup—beautifying herself. Whatever it took to look more attractive to men and feel better about herself. Meanwhile, she grew up listening to her dad make derogatory comments about women that made her feel uncomfortable. This combination of sexist messages and feeling she was never pretty enough greatly impacted her connection to her body, her sexual identity, and speaking her truth.

Sara first began to explore self-pleasuring as part of her therapeutic process. Over time, she became more in tune with what her body preferred. Eventually this reconnection to her body became an instrument for self-love. She told me in one of our sessions, "I have genuine love for my body now." Therapy and body connection became a way to heal and reconnect to her innate worth. It's amazing how tapping into the canvas of her own body, with its nooks and crannies and pleasure zones, became a medicine cabinet for her soul.

Eventually Sara started a relationship with a new guy. This time, she was more intentional about what *she* wanted and felt more confident saying it. After a couple months of dating, they had sex because she felt close to him, not because she needed proof that she was desirable as an ego boost. Exploring her boundaries with masturbation, as well engaging in psychotherapy and the stages of bodyfulness, were crucial to Sara owning her physical and emotional limits and understanding her motivations in a relationship.

~ 12 ~

Be a Humble Warrior

You must love in such a way that the other person feels free.
—Thich Nhat Hanh

I SAT WITH my client Roxy inside an office in the Castro District of San Francisco, hearing the train rattle up and down Market Street. It was the year 2000, and Roxy was a black transgender woman in her late thirties with the build of a linebacker. She'd always make a grand entrance to our sessions, not because of her size but because she arrived with a story and contagious laughter.

I was an intern with a clinic serving the LGBT community during graduate school. Given the greater awareness and inclusivity today for sexual identity, we might now say they serve the LGBTTQQIAAP community (lesbian, gay, bisexual, transgender, transsexual, queer, questioning, intersex, asexual, ally, pansexual). Having an interest in sexuality and infectious disease, specifically HIV/AIDS, I got to work with Roxy because she was HIV-positive.

Our time together was a window into the dysphoria she'd felt growing up in a male-assigned body. She told me about her anger toward the criminal justice system after spending years stuck in a male prison (for drug possession) despite identifying as female. At the end of our time together, Roxy commented that although she was used to being stared at, in therapy she felt seen for who she truly was.

I admired how Roxy, and only Roxy, decided how to inhabit her body. She embodied joy in the face of struggle, as seen in the way she adored—and adorned—her body. She had magnetic energy—often laughing, dancing, and dressing for a night out. Despite a lifetime of being imprisoned by expectations to identify and act like a man, Roxy lived in her body with freedom and full expression.

It was a time of possibility, thanks to recent advances in HIV/AIDS medicine. Many of my clients spent the 1990s preparing for the inevitable, viewing the diagnosis as a probable death sentence. They needed help reenvisioning the future they feared they might not have; it was about learning how to live, not preparing to die.

We all want to live fully—body-fully, pleasure-fully and relation-ally. And like Roxy, in our heart of hearts we want to be seen for who we truly are. Psychotherapy is intended to help do that. It's an intimate process of engaging with someone honestly to develop trust and awaken through the experience. The same can be said for deep relationships of any kind—family, friendship, and, of course, romantically intimate ones.

At this point in the book, hopefully you're becoming more intimate with your own badass, beautiful self. And hopefully you're feeling more tranquil in your body, equipped with some tools to manage life's inevitable ebb and flow of pain and pleasure. We've worked on connecting to the language of the body and ways to embody more self-regulation, sensuality, play, and pleasure. We've worked on how to own what you desire, feel deserving of it, and give yourself permission to receive it. Armed with all this self-awareness, you're primed to share in life's pleasures with a special someone, right? Maybe that's the reason you decided to read this book to begin with. After all, when most people see the word *pleasure* in a title, they think, "Must be a sex book!"

Instead I would say this book is ultimately about intimacy, a word that most people reduce to sex but it's actually about the *nonphysical* aspects of connection as well, such as emotional intimacy. Language is powerful, which is why it's helpful to understand the difference between sensuality, desire, intimacy, sex, and eroticism, especially if you care about having them in your life. I talked about sensuality in chapter 10; I explored desire in chapter 11; and now, for the next few chapters, we'll investigate how bodyfulness expands your capacity for intimacy and enhances pleasure in erotic relationships. Giddy up.

RELATIONSHIP OXYGEN

Vulnerability is the price of admission for most long-term meaningful relationships. Not the performative vulnerability we increasingly see on social media but the raw, shaky-voice, put-your-feelings-out-there kind of vulnerability. And yet it's challenging enough to be honest with ourselves—to face our self-doubts, quirky habits, and bizarre fantasies, let alone reveal them to someone else. We keep those skeletons in the closet for a reason. To our nervous system, there's little difference between the news of an HIV diagnosis and revealing a secret to someone; they can both register as potential threats. We fear our disclosures and confessions will lead to judgment, rejection, or being taken advantage of. Because let's get real—they sometimes do.

> All we really want is love's confusing joy.
> —*Rumi*

So why bother being vulnerable? Because humans are social creatures meant to bond with other sentient beings. We need one another like we need oxygen. Not only do we feel better when we're in this together, but our survival, in large part, depends on having a tribe that knows us and protects us. Validation and feedback from others are invaluable. Beyond survival, relationships add meaning, purpose, and sweetness; our pleasures and joys can expand when we share them with others. And if we're lucky, our chemistry with someone can ignite a pleasure unlike anything we've experienced alone.

The good news is bodyfulness helps you expand your capacity for intimacy, as you may have already discovered while exploring the inquiries in the previous chapters. Why? Because intimacy is "in-to-me-I-see," and bodyfulness gives you the opportunity to "see" yourself from the inside out. It comes from the Latin word *intimare*, which means "to press against or make familiar." This foundation of self-familiarity makes a big difference in relationships. Bodyfulness practices connect you to your heart and emotional body, awakening empathy, which can inspire bonding with others. Likewise, others can help you delight in your experience of bodyfulness; it's a two-way street.

RISK MANAGEMENT

What holds us back from sharing our pleasures with others? Life. Its hardships and heartaches can shut us off from our body and others. Like that old saying: once bitten, twice shy. Plus, the truth is—every sexual and romantic relationship ends until there's finally one that doesn't. In life, just like in all things pleasurable, we might be flying high one minute and face-plant the next. For all the pleasures intimate relationships bring, sometimes they can also lead to fumbling and fracturing.

I believe if you practice taking risks in other areas of your life, with your body, you'll be less afraid of doing so with your heart. I think of the time I was coming to the end of a trail race, bombing down the mountain with runner's high (an example of a pleasurable flow state), when I tripped and crashed into the bushes. I brushed myself off, thankful my teeth were intact (after braces, mouth guards, and gum replacement surgery, my mouth is worth a fortune.) Then I looked down and noticed my mangled finger. To this day I lose my grip with that hand, dropping things I'd normally never drop. It used to annoy me more but eventually I realized I had to make peace with my gangly finger. I decided it would be a reminder of the inevitable risk in saying yes to opportunities of all kinds despite potential injury. And I decided that it wasn't going to keep me from the exhilaration of doing more trail races.

What about you? What are the stories "written" on your body in the form of scars, breakages, injuries, or tattoos? What do they represent to you and how can you find meaning or a reminder in each of them?

Wisdom and courage come from lived experience. Not merely *thinking* about experiences. Not from reading a book. Not from sitting on the couch being mindful. It comes from getting off the couch and engaging with your body, engaging with others, and engaging with the world. Bodyfulness engages the inner world of your body dynamically with the outer world. It means being more aware of emotions, expanding your capacity to feel, love, and see the connectedness of people and the natural world. To fall in love with love itself, with your body, or anything really—an electrifying thunderstorm or a resplendent starry night—is to fully awaken. And yet the more tender and open we let our hearts be, the more exposed they are to pain.

The yoga teacher and author Seane Corn once said, "If you hurt that bad you must have loved that big." Falling in love is the epitome of vulnerability. We are showered in the pleasures of new-person energy, flooded with a cascade of bonding and excitatory hormones. Depending on the ride and if or how it ended, you could feel a trauma to your entire system; *heartache* is a literal term. As the Chinese philosopher Lao Tzu said, "Love is of all passions the strongest, for it attacks simultaneously the head, the heart, and the senses."

Even more challenging, our body has different agendas for recovery—the heart is *grieving* while the mind is busy *explaining* what happened, which, as we know, doesn't entirely work. Even if we logically understand why the relationship didn't work, our neurochemistry (especially the bonding hormone oxytocin) can keep us attached and in longing for weeks or months. This is why grief needs to release through the body—with tears, audible sound, gentle stretches of our connective tissue, movements to get blood flowing, containment with hugs, and unconditional compassion. We may never *get over* someone after a breakup, but we can get *through it* to love big again, and maybe even a little more wisely next time.

The alternative to loving big—being closed off emotionally and physically—comes with its own side effects such as regret, loneliness, and superficiality. My yoga teacher Jeffrey Bores would say, "You were never really in the pose to begin with unless you fell out of it." You can stay on the sidelines, skipping that challenging yoga pose, or the connection with a potential partner, but over time your world (and I dare say, your heart) gets smaller and smaller, smothered in your attempt to stay emotionally safe and in control.

Has your heart ever felt broken? If so, what did you notice in your body during that experience? How did you get through it? If not, were you never in "the pose" of the relationship to begin with, just *pose-ing* so you wouldn't get hurt? If you still grieve a broken heart, imagine ways to nurture your emotional body with kindness, rest, and release.

FROM STRENGTH WE CAN SURRENDER

Your relationship with your body helps ground you in the courage to be vulnerable in relationships. Armed with your bodyful toolbox, which supports you and gives you agency, you're better able to handle potential pain *and* be receptive to potential pleasures. Vulnerability is less intimidating when you come from a place of emotional and physical strength.

There's an old-school idea that being dominant is the measure of strength and being vulnerable is an indication of weakness. The irony is that the strongest person is actually someone who can let go—of their ego, of the need to be "right," of having power over others. The Humble Warrior yoga pose embodies this idea beautifully. Physically, your legs are in a Warrior 1 position—extended, strong and sturdy like the base of a mountain, while your upper body is open and deferential. Your hands are clasped behind your back, your chest expanded and lifted, and you bend forward with your head toward your bent knee in front of you. The gesture of bowing from the position of a warrior illustrates that *from strength we can surrender.*

Listening to and engaging your body—with embodied mindfulness, awareness of your nervous system, interoception, and subtle body energy—helps you be that strong-yet-kind warrior within. To hold opposing or multiple feelings and attitudes within you at once may not be easy but it's a sure sign of emotional maturity. If you want genuine connection, to care and be cared for, to love and be loved, then embody your tenderness *and* your strength like that of a humble warrior.

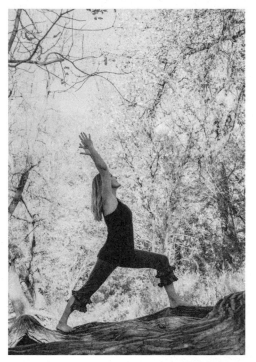

Warrior 1

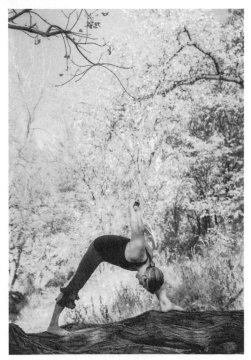

Humble Warrior

Naturally things get more complicated once we add another human body into the mix. Relationships have a way of leading us straight to our wounds, with the opportunity to repeat them or heal them. They can be repairing, literally helping you repair old childhood wounds and body memory, by cultivating new relationships that are reliable and supportive.

There are lots of factors that influence our ability to feel the pleasures of relationships, especially the stickier ones that are sexual and erotic. I've touched upon some of these already, and it would take a tome to cover them all. But I'll briefly share a couple important theories regarding what blocks us from receiving the healthy pleasures that relationships can bring.

ATTACHMENT THEORY

After college I worked in a university psychiatry department in a study on childhood attachment. We replicated the infamous "Strange Situation" experiment, meant to observe how young children respond to the temporary absence of a parent and how it might predict future relationship styles. I played the role of "stranger," and the funniest—or perhaps creepiest—part was that my uniform was a black sheet over my entire body and a gas mask over my face. The parent would leave the room and I'd walk in, like something out of a zombie movie, while my colleagues watched from the other side of a two-way mirror. The kids who cried at the sight of me were thought to be more *insecurely attached*, while the kids who looked puzzled for a moment but merely went back to their toys were thought to be more *securely attached*.

Just as predicted by attachment science, contact with a loving, responsive partner is a powerful buffer against danger and threat. When we change our love relationships, we change our brains and change our world.
—Sue Johnson

Researchers agree that a big influence on our adult relationships is the "attachment styles" we developed with caregivers as children. The different types—*secure, anxious, avoidant,* and *disorganized*—in large part determine whether we trust people to meet our needs and not harm us; be there for us, but not smother us. While many factors play a role in our relationship choices as adults, including genes and other environmental experiences throughout our life, these attachment categories provide a helpful map of how and whom we love—because neither the how nor the who is random. Understanding these styles is part of your embodied mindfulness practice, that first stage of bodyfulness, because it expands your self-awareness. It helps you better understand the connection and feedback loops between your emotional reactions, trauma held in your body from past relationships, how you repeat patterns, and the importance of being with people who co-regulate you.

Securely attached adults tend to be stable emotionally. They have more emotional intelligence, which is defined as having self-awareness, self-regulation, empathy, and social skills. They value being honest and engage equally with their partner. Securely attached people aren't immune to relationship problems but they are more likely to not over-personalize the circumstance. Those with *anxious* attachment are so afraid of being alone and tend to look to the other person to save or complete them. They can be clingy and overreact to their partner's absence, perceiving it as abandonment.

With *avoidant* attachment, people can be distant, aloof, and shut down emotionally. They tend to focus on their independence or they're so afraid of closeness that they don't even bother trying. Either way, they want to keep their feelings subdued and deny their subconscious needs for closeness but often aren't able to, so they can be prone to emotional storms. People who have *disorganized* attachment most likely experienced chaos and abuse growing up. They tend to be abusive and rageful, and they lack empathy. It's worth noting that people can vacillate between an anxious and avoidant style depending on the person they have as a partner.

These unhealthy relationship patterns you modeled growing up can become stuck body memories and mental beliefs, ingrained by time. Then as an adult, if you come across someone who treats you in a similar dynamic to the caregiver(s) who most influenced your wounds, you might regress to your childlike self, having knee-jerk reactions in the ways I just mentioned, or even pursue them as a partner in a subconscious attempt to resolve your childhood trauma. It's confusing, if not impossible, for anyone to know how to cope until they engage in psychotherapy and do regular, intentional work to regulate themselves, and practice agency and self-compassion.

Check out the Head, Heart, Gut, Groin Moving Meditation in the appendix on page 277. Once you have finished the meditation, contemplate the "viewpoints" of those four layers that influence your decision-making in relationships. For example, your head might say, "I want too much from a partner," while your heart says, "I want to be chosen and cared for." Your gut churns, "This person isn't available," while your groin chimes in with, "I want to be desired." This helps you understand the different parts of yourself and explore ways to integrate them as you make decisions.

DISTANCER-PURSUER DYNAMIC

Here's an example that connects attachment styles with the first two stages of bodyfulness. When you've got two insecurely attached people in a relationship it creates an addictive pattern. A common example of this is the distancer-pursuer dynamic, found when someone with avoidant attachment pairs with someone with anxious attachment. Someone with an avoidant relationship style tends to *deal but not feel*. They might be in a constant state of hyperarousal, going through the motions of life but never releasing or expressing their feelings. This person is the *distancer*, who tends to respond to relationship stress, and even intimacy, by moving away from their partner. They want physical and emotional distance because they have difficulty with vulnerability.[1] This person could likely benefit from learning embodied mindfulness and healthier *discharge* strategies.

On the other hand, someone with an anxious relationship style tends to *feel but not deal*; their feelings can be like a roller coaster, but they don't learn how to manage and express them effectively. They tend to become the *pursuer*, responding to relationship stress by seeking discussion, togetherness, and expression. They are quick to try to fix what they think is wrong and feel anxious about the distance their partner has created, taking it personally. This individual could benefit from learning embodied mindfulness and healthier, more appropriate *containment* strategies. Neither of these styles of relating is pleasurable or satisfying, and if they're paired together it's going to be a bumpy ride: a push-pull dynamic.

The drama that ensues creates excitatory chemicals in the brain (endorphins) and a body in a fight-flight-freeze mode of adrenaline bursts, which oddly can keep people hooked in their discontent. Oh, how these cycles repeat themselves and provoke us when we're not conscious of them.

Another common pattern I see connected to insecure attachment is chasing unavailable people. For example, my client Sherri came to me because she was with a man who supported her emotionally, but she felt smothered. Even though she wanted someone kind and stable, that was an unfamiliar dynamic because she had always been with unavailable men. One of the curious things we humans do is push away things or people we want or need simply because they are unfamiliar. Sherri was used to "the chase" in relationships, and when that didn't happen, she got kinda bored. If she actually "caught" the guy, she felt validated; it proved she was so special because she was able to captivate someone. This was all unconscious, of course. Since the relationships she was chasing never lasted because they weren't emotionally mature, Sherry continually felt wounded.

In therapy we realized this was similar to her dynamic with her dad, who was inconsistent and often unavailable. As an adult she derived excitement from *eroticizing* rejection: the chase maintained the belief that she had to *earn* a man's love. The teachings of the first stage of bodyfulness helped her slow down to viscerally notice her chain reaction toward the "bad boy" and how it was a by-product of old wounds. We practiced noticing where in her body she would get set off and then we engaged the second stage of bodyfulness with breath, grounding movements, and healing self-touch to soothe the triggered areas of her body and nervous system. We paired this with discussions on self-love and self-nurturance (including the tending and befriending I mentioned in chapter 5). We also explored other ways to feed her dopamine-craving brain and body through adventurous hobbies (lively pleasures) rather than seeking it from unavailable man-childs.

You might mentally have an idea of what a healthy relationship looks like, but you won't *live it* until you viscerally experience the ease of a relationship with a securely attached person. That kind of relationship might seem boring at first (you were used to things being tumultuous) but as you become more bodyful—with self-awareness, accountability, better boundaries—you grow tired of toxic dynamics. This is freedom. The attachment psychologist Diane Poole Heller said, "As we familiarize ourselves more with secure attachment, our relationships become easier and more rewarding—we're less reactive, more receptive, more available for connection, healthier, and much more likely to bring out the securely attached in others."[2] And it's more likely to come your way once you've unfolded into the third stage of bodyfulness.

These unhealthy relationships dynamics do not have to be a life sentence. During the first stage of bodyfulness you can better understand why you react the way you do by making the unconscious more conscious, with kindness, starting in the body where the old traumas first got stuck. In the second stage you can practice managing, modulating, and hopefully replacing those reactive patterns with healthier behaviors. You begin to trust yourself more and this helps you live from the third stage of bodyfulness. Here you can channel your inner Aretha as she sang about R-E-S-P-E-C-T.

DIFFERENTIATION: SEPARATELY TOGETHER

That first stage of bodyfulness is a process of being self-aware but also being self-accountable—you own your shit, not someone else's. This is again about boundaries and recognizing what is and is not your responsibility, whether it be apologizing for buying the wrong item at the grocery store (taking responsibility) or not overreacting to your coworkers temper tantrum (not taking responsibility). Someone else's physical, mental, or emotional experience is theirs, and you have yours. Between self-awareness and awareness of "other," there is space to be a *compassionate witness*, instead of taking responsibility for the other person's feelings. Sure, we have influence over people's feelings, but that doesn't mean we are ultimately responsible for their perspective. There is a big difference.

The psychiatrist David Schnarch calls this idea *differentiation*. It describes the ability to balance your individual identity with the coupling of a relationship. You have a healthy sense of being separate and unique while still able to care for the well-being of the other person as best you can. You recognize that your partner is an adult, responsible for their own feelings and actions. You certainly sway each other, but you're still separate individuals. When people in a relationship are differentiated, they have healthy boundaries and expectations and less drama. This holds true for parent-child relationships as well. Bodyfulness encourages differentiation because it's a practice of grounding in your own internal experience on a regular basis, not becoming overly involved or taking complete responsibility for someone else's.

TWO KINDS OF INTIMACY

I once asked a client if she felt more comfortable with physical or emotional intimacy. She said physical, because emotional intimacy "can be used against me." Sadly, her tendency to be emotionally distant was depriving others the pleasure of knowing her awesomeness, and her to know theirs. Physical and emotional intimacy are not easy for most people; relationships and sex have become even more disembodied. All the more challenging, two people can be mismatched in a relationship—one person feeling more comfortable with physical intimacy, while the other person feels more comfortable with emotional intimacy. Ask yourself, "Which one (if any) am I more comfortable with?"

You might avoid emotional intimacy yet still yearn for it in your heart. Some of the things my clients have told me they want from a romantic partner include: feeling emotionally supported, feeling safe to authentically expressing themselves, having unconditional acceptance, getting honest and constructive feedback, and sharing a sense of humor.

I've touched on some of these already in the book, so I'll elaborate more on the pleasures of physical intimacy, since sexual and erotic pleasure have been so dysfunctional in the US. The obstacles to healthy physical intimacy are many, but the main issues include: low libido, different levels of desire, generally blah sex that's always the same ("Groundhog Day sex"), performance anxiety, losing attraction, sexual trauma, problems regarding porn use, wanting to explore polyamory, adultery, fertility problems, and issues around sexual identity. As you can see, there's a lot that might feel confusing as you open your heart or body to someone else.

Most people would probably agree that being naked is as "exposed" and vulnerable as you get. One of my clients felt that there was something wrong with her for wanting the lights out sometimes while undressing with her partner. For all my talk about feeling at home in your body, it's normal to have days or even longer phases where you're *not* feeling sexy or open to sharing yourself. Perhaps you're sleep deprived, have a work deadline, are enduring a loss, or the ceviche you ate didn't agree with you. When I asked her, "What if it were *okay* to not feel comfortable naked sometimes?" I saw the tightness in her chest soften in relief.

Now, if your body is *always* something you hide you certainly won't be savoring it with someone else. This is why bodyfulness is such an important foundation to enjoying intimacy of all kinds. When you can listen and receive what the relationship brings up, breath by breath, with self-compassion and a body you respect—physically, emotionally, and energetically—you can better ride the wave.

To be clear, sex doesn't need to be intimate to be necessary or enjoyable. It's okay to have times when you don't have the bandwidth for an intimate relationship—emotionally or physically—because you're dealing with other important matters. Sometimes you need space. Sometimes you get bored. Sometimes your passion is focused on a project. Sometimes you might think, "Forget intimacy, I just want to get laid." Sometimes you want to be animalistic. It's natural to have times when you don't have energy for a deep emotional experience and you would just rather "get it in." Similar to how we need a variety of food groups and movements to be balanced and bodyful, we need different types of physical intimacy over our lifetime. Once in a while you just want to go to McDonald's—get in and out quickly. As long as you're aware, honest, and considerate with others about where you're it, I would argue that it's all fair game.

SEXUAL SEEKERS

Americans may be repressed as a culture overall but most of us still *want* to think of ourselves as sexual throughout our life spans. Because Americans are competitive and attached to our youth, we end up being "seekers" when it comes to improving our sex lives.

The problem is there are so many misconceptions that interfere with people's erotic pleasures. What we need is some *sexual intelligence.* This is about noticing and correcting false beliefs around sex, pleasure, and physical intimacy over time. It's about dropping the belief that sex will always be tidy and go as "planned." It's not a fairy tale that hides the less glamorous realities such as bad breath, painful sex, problems with incontinence, and old people getting it on. Sex involves body fluids, naked bodies with injuries, and messed-up sheets. Condoms break, people get infections, and klutzy moments happen.

Sexual intelligence recognizes we inhabit bodies that are aging and require us to adapt. As the novelist Erica Jong said, "Sex doesn't disappear, it just changes forms."[3] Seems baby boomers feel the same way: the greatest increase in sexually transmitted infections between 2014 and 2017 occurred among people over age sixty, increasing by 23 percent, which is proof that they're still getting after it, albeit not very safely.[4]

Sexual intelligence is also about not comparing our sex lives to other people's sex lives. No one knows what's going on behind the closed doors of other people's relationships—even the two people in one can have totally different versions. We idealize others' relationships based on limited information, such as their social media pictures and pronouncements.

The actual reality of people's sex lives may surprise you. The next time you think the neighbors are having earth-shattering sex all the time, here's what's going on according to a 2017 study in the *Archives of Sexual Behavior*:

- The average adult has sex 54 times a year.
- The average sexual encounter lasts about 30 minutes.
- People in their twenties have sex more than 80 times per year.
- People in their forties have sex about 60 times a year.
- Sex drops to 20 times per year by age sixty-five.
- People born in the 1990s (millennials) had sex the least often.
- The typical married person has sex an average of 51 times a year.
- "Very happy" couples have sex, on average, 74 times a year.
- Active people have more sex (that's what I'm talking about).[5]

Those may be the stats, but the actual lived reality of your erotic life gets to be whatever you decide it to be.

COMMUNICATION, THE BEDROCK TO MAKE YOUR BED ROCK

As a therapist trying to help couples realize and share their wants for pleasure, I believe that communication is the name of the game. Sadly, we have more ways to communicate than ever and yet we've never been worse at it. For example, research has shown that large proportions of Americans don't even tell their partner when sex hurts.[6] They'd rather suffer in silence. There's a saying that we're only as sick as our secrets, which hold centuries of systemic repression and trauma. But I'll let you in on my own secret: it's liberating to be honest.

Do you know in your head what pleasures you want but then it comes out as gibberish when you try to ask for it? For many people, self-disclosure is awkward and scary. But according to the sex and relationship columnist Dan Savage, gay men don't beat around the bush; when they meet, it typically starts with some variation of these four words: "What are you into?" Direct, confident, clear. Whatever your erotic preferences, one thing is true: *you can't receive the pleasure you don't ask for!*

"I WANT, I NEED, I FEEL"

A friend was doing video calls with her partner while in the early stages of a long-distance relationship. One night he pointed out that she tended to move her tongue along the corners of her mouth and teeth somewhat salaciously. She had no idea and was embarrassed. Like the friend who doesn't point out the kale in your teeth, he could have easily not said anything.

Which is what many people do, but with much bigger consequences than feeling awkward about a mouth tick. One client's wife revealed she was ending the marriage because "I haven't loved you for the past decade." Mind blown. Another client's boyfriend ended things by telling him, "Our sex is too vanilla." It was the first time he'd mentioned it, giving my client no opportunity to course correct. We aren't mind readers, for crying out loud.

Honesty really is the best policy. I once saw street art in Cuba that translated to "The truth hurts. The lies kill. But the doubt tortures." We torture each other by withholding our feelings, and we end up causing more pain in the long run.

Why have you avoided telling someone the truth? The most common reasons I hear are that they fear conflict and that they don't want to hurt someone's feelings, jeopardize the relationship, be disliked, or be ignored. So instead, they convince themselves their issue isn't valid; they obsess in their head or to others instead of the actual person; they keep it to themselves and then feel resentful, grumpy, or get passive-aggressive; they rationalize it, shut down, or create some other sort of nonrelated conflict.

The word *conflict* needs a PR agent. We should associate it with resolution and closure through transparency and acknowledgment, with the chance to get closer to each other. My high school history teacher wanted us to think about tests as opportunities to grow, so he called them "OTEs" (opportunities to excel). Let's apply this renaming to conflict. Unless someone has an avoidant or defiant personality (such as narcissism), disagreements can be OTRs (opportunities to resolve)—ways to deepen your bond. Research indicates that gay and lesbian couples are fairer and use fewer tactics to control the other person or be hostile in a disagreement. Perhaps this is because they show more affection and humor when they argue, making them more likely to remain positive after an argument.[7] Just remember that honesty without compassion can be cruel, while compassion without honesty can do harm. Read that sentence again.

How comfortable are you asking for what you want outside of the bedroom? If you can't be direct about how you like your coffee, you'll probably struggle to say how you like your foreplay. (And remember, foreplay begins the moment your last encounter ended.) Next time you're picking dinner restaurants or upholstery, practice stating your preference. Keep working at it until you ask for what you want with more gusto and confidence (which is different from arrogance). The psychologist Jack Morin talked about being ruthless in asking for what you want erotically, not in the context of being sadistic and overly selfish but in reaching out and taking in your desires unapologetically.[8]

The relationship therapist Esther Perel explains there are seven key verbs that we should all keep in mind when communicating with a partner: ask, give, receive, take, imagine/play, share, refuse.[9] To *ask* means to request what you want and need; to *give* means to be generous in giving pleasure and joy to others; to *receive* means to accept anything from compliments to gifts to sexual touch; to *take* means to empower yourself to identify what feels good and pursue it; to *imagine* means to share yourself and your fantasies playfully and creatively; to *share* means to interact in ways that feel bonding; to *refuse* means stating what doesn't feel good and having boundaries.

Looking over these verbs, which of them are you most comfortable with? Which ones are you the least comfortable with? In what areas might you need to say no or yes?

Silence also speaks volumes. Your body language makes up for what your words don't express. Eye rolls, fidgeting, nervous laughter, and a clenched jaw convey a lot, but it's unproductive. These types of passive or passive-aggressive styles just delay getting to the point. Clear, direct communication that starts with "I want," "I need," and "I feel" is the tried-and-true method. It's about being curious, not critical. No one is going to respond well to accusations, but they'll probably respond well to your genuine and heartfelt experience.

~ 13 ~

Magnetic Intimacy

The heart has reasons of which the mind knows nothing.
—*Blaise Pascal*

SEX, THE GOOD OL' AMERICAN WAY, is done during a proper time (married adults, procreating) and a proper place (at home, in bed, in the dark). It has been *mechanical, performative,* and *productive.* The problem? These ways of thinking about sex interfere with our body connection and our bond to the other person—two profoundly intimate pleasures. This chapter redefines sex in a bodyful way as *energetic, authentic,* and an experiential *process* to be shared. Let's compare:

Mechanical. This is how you do it: In both sex education and sex therapy, the focus has been on the *mechanics,* as if we were machines. Professionals have spoken of things such as refractory periods, the size and insertion of anatomy into orifices, and how sperm and egg unite. It's like an episode of *Science Friday:* "Do this. Then that. And now pretend it never happened." Slam, bam; thank you, ma'am. Bodyfulness doesn't limit sexual pleasure to genitals shoved into people's holes; it's more than merely PIV (penis-in-vagina) penetration. How your body functions is just one small aspect of physical intimacy. The sacred side of sex means inhabiting your body and breathing alongside the breath of another, your presence with each other an act of energy exchange.

Performative. This is how it should look: Sexual pleasure is for the young and able-bodied. Bonus points if you're wearing lingerie or other accoutrements and impress your lover with acrobatic positions. You're the observer from the outside looking in, double-checking that you're doing it "right." One more opportunity to evaluate yourself. You hope they like your "show" enough to have an encore someday. Sex is evaluated by how long it lasts, how hard or wet the genitals are, and how many times someone's orgasmed. A distracted mind focused on performance is a pleasure killer. Bodyfulness, in contrast, sees sexual pleasure as much more than a step-by-step in a *Cosmo* article or how it's portrayed in a soap opera.

Productive. This is why you do it: Sex should lead to an orgasm or conception, otherwise what's the point? You've failed at sex if you didn't both "achieve" an orgasm. Or if someone did have an orgasm but it happened too soon, took too long, or left the other person behind. This all-or-nothing attitude implies that penetration equals sex. (Although throngs of folks raised in abstinence-based religions might beg to differ. My favorite is the Mormon concept of "soaking," which means a man sticks his penis in a vagina but doesn't move it around, therefore it somehow doesn't count as sex. Gimme a break.) Various different types of touch, such as caressing, kissing or massaging, are not part of the equation. After all, who has time for such frivolity? And besides, lingering in foreplay or the afterglow may indicate that a couple likes sex a little *too* much. Bodyfulness lets go of the goal-oriented mindset (as you practiced with sensuality, playfulness, and liveliness), seeing sex as a chance for exploration—just for the pure pleasure of it.

These examples remove people from their bodily and relational experience. We might as well engage in virtual-reality sex. If we strip away these crusty old viewpoints and engage in sex bodyfully, we are channeling our *energy* and *authenticity* within an experiential *process*.

Energetic. Typically, erotic energy is used interchangeably with sexual energy. But the word *erotic* derives from the Greek God Eros, who celebrated the love of life with fervor. Ancient Greeks saw eros energy as a passionate and powerful life-force energy that expressed itself in many ways, not just sexually. Eros energy was about immersing yourself in your experiences with abandon, whether it be a surge of emotion at a sporting event or the exultation of jumping into a tide pool. Erotic energy is a process of awakening rather than shutting down, and it can lead to pleasure states. Erotic pleasure emerges from a connection to your physicality, your felt sense, your emotions, and the charge of energy shared with someone else. Giving and receiving energy with another is essential to your aliveness. Eroticism and sexual pleasure are part of the natural flow of life's energy, your own life-force energy, and being human. By limiting or ignoring this in your life, you're limiting and ignoring your vitality, essentially deadening your senses.

Authentic. Our sexuality is as unique as our fingerprints. You can "do" sex, perform for your date or partner (the facade), or you can inhabit yourself from *within* the experience (being real). When we naturally express ourselves from the inside out, our essence can radiate. This freedom from being overly self-conscious—respecting where you're at on your journey and not merely accepting yourself but loving yourself—can inspire others.

An experiential process. We chase after the goalpost of life—whether it be the promise of the next best thing or an orgasm. We think that's what will make us happy, but I believe we take more pleasure in the *quest* than the conquest. The poet David Whyte agrees: "Our human essence lies not in arrival but in being almost there. We are creatures who are on the way, our journey a series of impending anticipated arrivals."[1] Anticipation is a powerful hook. Erotic energy is a cocktail of excited anxiety and relaxation. Obstacles are key to erotic tension: "When will I see her?" "What makes him tick?" "Will he touch me farther up my thigh?" We love the tempting, teasing buildup of foreplay, we've just been too busy to give it the time and energy it deserves.

In which case, I've got good news: you've been engaging in the ultimate foreplay *throughout the entire book*. Those moments of play, diverse movement, sweating, breathing, and flowing have primed you for the erotic pleasures you choose. Because sex is presence. Sex is sensuality. Sex is creativity. Sex is being immersed. Sex is a flow state. Sex is relaxation. Sex is relaxed excitement. It's not rocket science to see how engaging your body in different ways throughout the previous chapters sows the seeds for erotic pleasure. Now let's give them some water to blossom in your relationships.

FOUR LOVE MYTHS

In the first section of the book, I talked about the messed-up messages we heard about our bodies and sex. Well, we've also been lied to about love, in ways that interfere with healthy relationship pleasure. The standard heteronormative narrative in the US fed us fairy tales about romantic relationships, leaving us with a narrow definition about love and unrealistic expectations about what's acceptable. Let me dispel four myths that cause us more pain than pleasure:

Myth 1: Love Heals All

Love has the power to redeem or rescue you, and the power of your love heals a damaged person. *Nope.* Someone else's love alone cannot "fix" you. (First of all, you are not broken.) Nor can your love fix them. It's a bit egotistical to think we could even be that magical. Just as we have to recognize our own potential and the potential of love, we have to recognize our own limits and the limits of love.

We all need close relationships, but those relationships need to be with people who can nurture us in return. If you are capable of giving love, you need to be with someone capable of loving you in return. Of course, no relationship is perfect; there can be a sprinkling of dysfunction in even the healthiest ones. But if you think your love will cure the deep, dark wounds in someone else—when they aren't willing to do the work of self-development—you'll likely be disappointed. Instead you're creating a toxic dynamic. I'm not dissing the power of love and, as I'll share in the next section, love for the sake of it in the spiritual sense is phenomenal and healing.

Myth 2: There Is One Soul Mate for You, and Your Quest Is to Find Them

Possible, but doubtful. Rarely can one person can be your everything. I interviewed a longtime matchmaker at LA Singles who said that clients come in with a ridiculously detailed list of expectations. It can be about status ("I'm looking for a Persian man at least ten years older than me.") or novelty ("I can't possibly date anyone from my own religion or race.") For some, it's geographic—they'll only date someone who lives in their part of town. People want to find their soul mate as if they're at a salad bar—a little of this ingredient, a little of that topping, dressing on the side. Getting clear on what you want is one thing but expecting salad bars to contain all your idiosyncratic ingredients is another.

I've heard dating coaches preach that making a highly detailed list of what you want from a suitor will lead to finding that perfect match. But a list that doesn't leave room for an actual human—neuroses, dissimilar preferences, crow's feet, and all—sets you up for exasperation. For some, their list is a reflection of (a) trying to find someone who looks so good on paper, it elevates their own status (arm candy). The ego looking for an Adonis to fill an emptiness within you or fill the role of the partner you think you're supposed to have; or (b) having an insatiable desire for the unconventional, found in other people who might be exhilarating for a while but aren't relationship material. This can be a blast, as long as both people are ready for the ride but will most likely crash and burn eventually.

Incidentally, fewer people are choosing to seek long-term partners these days anyway, much less a soul mate. In 1950, 78 percent of the population in the United States were married, while in 2014, more than 50 percent of the population identified as single.[2] Increasingly, people aren't interested in getting married or even having long-term relationships. They want the pleasures of sex and companionship—whether it be a friend with benefits or live-in lover—but they don't want to bother with the stodgy institution of marriage or the guarantee of a soul mate.

Myth 3: Be Selfless in Love and Sex; Don't Focus on Yourself

Conversely, *be self-full*. There's an old romantic story line that we should lose ourselves to our beloved. Please don't do that. Here's why: it's important to distinguish between sharing yourself—which is bonding and empathetic—and losing your identity to someone else's needs, which leads to codependency, anxious attachment, or later resentment.

Honor your selfish desires. I love this idea from the sex therapist and author Stella Resnick: When people compromise what they want, no one is all that happy. Ironically, once we do get what we want, it's natural to want to give back. So let's give to our partner because it feels good—out of generosity, not out of compromise. In the ancient yogic and Buddhist texts, there's a concept called *sympathetic joy*—the act of being happy for another's happiness. When we delight in our lover's success, it's not a sign of selfless love but soulful connection. Asking for what you want, paradoxically, creates a deeper bond within a relationship. Tantric philosophy agrees and also believes that giving women erotic satisfaction is of the utmost importance, leading to happier households and communities, one matriarch at a time. Here here!

Your desires shouldn't depend on someone else igniting them. They need to start with you. Erotic pleasure relies on feeling that *you* matter and that receiving your desires matter. So generate your erotic preferences and let your partner get to know this side of you. And don't rely on their reflection of you or their ability to fulfill your wants as the measure of whether you're desire worthy—see it in *yourself*. Sure, being the object of their desire is tantalizing for them, but let that hotness circulate within you whether they're around to reflect it back to you or not.

Myth 4: Long-Term Relationships Are the Epitome of Intimacy

Yes, and. Some multidecade relationships are examples of deep emotional and physical intimacy, while some are just two roommates bickering at each other for years. This emphasis on longevity as the gold standard is tired. Long-term relationships are not inherently better than shorter relationships, even though that's what most of us have been led to believe. This notion makes everyone who is *not* in a multidecade relationship feel that there's something wrong with them. And there isn't.

I understand both worlds. There was a time when I happened to be unattached and my friend called me out: "Shouldn't you be in some fabulous relationship given what you do for a living?" I couldn't help but laugh at his candor. I get it. You go to a personal trainer who looks fit, a financial planner who looks moneyed, and a relationship therapist who has a lifelong relationship. Whatever the profession, you want them to have their shit together, otherwise why would you be paying them?

I am not an expert on monogamy-till-death-do-us-part, and I've never claimed to be one. I am a *pleasure expert.* But I will say this: I've been fascinated by relationships throughout my career and have studied the different theories about what tethers us and why it matters. I've even done my own "field research" on the topic leading to lots of learning along the way. I've been married and I've been engaged (yes, to two different people). I've had eight-week, eight-month, and eight-year relationships. I've been drawn to people I met in my hometown but also in places as far away as Belize and Hawaii. I've experienced the new and exciting, the long and drawn out, the one-hit wonders, the old flames revisited, the too-good-to-be trues, the players, the nerds by day and nymphos by night . . . you get the point. Just as you wouldn't want to hire a trainer who is chiseled from lucky genes rather than the hard work of exercise, you don't want a relationship therapist who hasn't put themselves out there in the world of relationships.

My response to him was that I've had phases when I was un-coupled because I was either too young to know better or because I chose to leave something that felt unhealthy. I see people trudging through bad relationships for three main reasons: kids, finances, and the fear of being alone. With so much emphasis on being partnered in our culture, people fear being single more than they fear the pain of staying in something extinct (even though they might be quite lonely in the partnership anyway). And often when people do leave, they immediately jump into another relationship. I encourage the moments *between* relationships as pivotal times to reset and reconnect to yourself. It can help you eventually find someone who's capable of holding your heart when the time is right.

Staying together forever has equaled success, and uncoupling has equaled failure. I had a client who felt such shame after giving everything she had to a ten-year relationship. How was it a failure if she grew and surrendered to loving someone for a whole decade? It's like my friend who runs hundred-mile ultramarathons. He once collapsed at mile ninety-four and couldn't finish the race and was depressed for months afterward. Even though he ran a whopping *ninety-four miles*! May we all recognize the potential injury of staying in the "race" too long, because sometimes walking away is healthy and wise.

Our culture encourages married coupledom through tax breaks and shared health insurance, leaving many people trapped in marital "arrangements." I worry about the folks unhappily stuck with each other in silence. If we could share our feelings about the challenges of long-term relationships more openly, we'd be able to support one another and feel less ashamed. Of course, there are many happy, healthy long-term relationships out there—those just aren't the people who come to me for therapy!

There isn't one model for finding pleasure in a relationship, and the old model has broken down at the side of the road. Look beyond the standard paradigm because it's possible to experience the pleasures of intimacy from many kinds of connections and commitments. If we didn't associate uncoupling with failure, and if we weren't so afraid of being alone, we'd free ourselves from lifeless commitments. Your nonconformity—whether it be your relationship with a partner or with your body—might make others uncomfortable, but that is their problem, not yours. *You* get to decide what "success" means to you. So live and love in ways that work for you, not how others have said your relationship, sexuality, or body *should* look like.

RELATIONSHIPS AS SPIRITUAL PRACTICE

For years I proclaimed to my friends I was never going to get a tattoo because I didn't like pain or commitment. How could I possibly pick one image and one area of my body to stick with forever? I figured I'd wait until I turned sixty-five to take the plunge (fewer years to live with a tattoo I regretted). Commitment is easier when it's a hypothetical far away.

I ended up getting a tattoo in Leon, Nicaragua, twenty years ahead of time. I chose the optical phenomenon called the *green flash*. It happens on rare occasions after a sunset on a clear day over a distinct edge, such as the flat horizon of the ocean. It's caused by light refracting into the atmosphere; water vapor absorbs the yellow and orange light. Like a rainbow, the right conditions come together and there it is, a pleasant surprise. When I look down at the multicolored triangle with a green base surrounding the scar on my left foot, it's a reminder to honor all that is greater than myself.

Like the green flash, connection with someone else (whether it be erotic or nurturing energy) evokes something greater than you. Social bonds of all kinds are powerful. What if you approached your relationships (shorter ones, longer ones, not-forever ones) as spiritual experiences? As the psychiatrist Judith Orloff said, "Sexuality and spirit are intimately related. When you surrender sexually, you enter an open intuitive state, permitting the force of creation to flow through you, similar to how artists are moved."[3]

The meditation teacher Phillip Moffitt writes about relationships falling into three categories: transactional, egoic, or spiritual.[4] Transactional is about what you can *get* from the other person (financial security, children); egoic is about your partner helping to raise your status (they're hot, or have clout, so that gives *you* street cred too); whereas spiritual is about the person being your teacher. They inspire you to awaken and own your blind spots. Compassion and nonjudgmental awareness in any relationship is certainly not always easy but can be transformational in the best possible way. Moffitt compares it to a lifelong yoga or meditation practice—each day is a choice to step on the mat or sit on the cushion with integrity.

Whether it be a thirty-year monogamous relationship or a spring fling, if you are consciously curious about the experience, there can always be revelatory moments. Let whatever type of relationship you're in, and the gaps between them, be opportunities to expand. Even two ships passing in the night can be a jump-start for self-reflection. Listen with the first stage of bodyfulness to what reverberates in you—such as how your partner isn't "making" you feel a certain way but rather stirring the pot of something already stewing in you. Once we take responsibility, we can take agency.

The third stage of bodyfulness channels the tantric idea of bringing sweetness to all aspects of life and relationship moments, even the more mundane ones. Start by bringing your spiritual or creative energy to the day-to-day. Imagine how you can be more tender and thoughtful . . . or wilder and more undomesticated.

DATING AS PLEASURABLE?

After two promising dates, the only time Seema heard from Carlos was the occasional text at bar close asking, "You up?" Susan slept with a guy on their fourth date and he left a shit smear in her bed, then never messaged again. ("He really left his mark on me," she half-joked, half-lamented.) Ricardo ended a first date with a kiss so sloppy he needed a burping cloth.

Dating can be quite an ordeal, when many people just want the real deal. All those screens instead of live interactions lead some people to forget that a human deserving respect is on the other side. It's far different from meeting organically—as neighbors or colleagues; in intentional communities, such as clubs, camps, retreats, and educational experiences that bond people through common ground and shared experience.

Too often people measure potential compatibility based on a bathroom selfie, spending two seconds per image. One of my friends in his early thirties had an age range from barely legal (eighteen) to fossil (one hundred, the age limit). It was all a joke to him. As the comedian Shani Silver said, "Somewhere along the internet we decided to adopt a form of dating so lazy that it requires little more than the joint of your right thumb to participate. . . . A passionless process where we barely have to think, much less develop feelings."[5]

I am fascinated by the cultural differences for what is acceptable body expression in people's online photos. One friend went home to Nigeria and noticed the pictures of women were focused on bodily curves and sex appeal. When he traveled to Japan the next month he noticed women's pictures were photos of mountains, flowers, or large groups of people, as a way to hide themselves. Talk about preserving the mystery.

I've helped clients challenge another cultural myth: that if they are struggling with dating, (or *any* relationship, whether it be romantic, work, or parenting) it means they're *simply not trying hard enough.* Quite the contrary. Many were trying plenty hard but doing so within a culture that doesn't help foster genuine relationships. In this era of "me, me, me," *narcissism* has become a real buzzword. It's the relationship kryptonite of our time, characterized by a lack of empathy, exerting control over others, disconnecting from feelings in order to get ahead, and prioritizing self-interests at the expense of others. Amid all the fake news and fake implants, we need empathy and honesty more than ever, on and off the dating apps.

How can this search for a companion be more pleasurable, given the pretty painful tales out there? See it as a marathon, not a sprint, requiring perseverance and a sense of humor. Equipped with your inner toolbox of listening, release/containment methods, and owning what you want, dating bodyfully helps you handle the tumultuous ride. For my client Denise, we worked on trusting her body's messages and intuition to discern the securely attached folks from the players. What was her gut instinct telling her, based on verbal and nonverbal communication? And how could she recognize and reorient her body's responses (given the nervous system can react like it's reliving past stress)? I helped her to be more aware of her emotional chain reaction in order to stay viscerally regulated and prevent overthinking, which is all too common with matters of the heart. Through breathing, diverse movement, and nurturing thoughts and self-touch, Denise made movement her medicine by exercising prior to a date and even having the date be an activity to keep things flowing, literally and figuratively.

The playful pleasure exercises in this book can help you with three important aspects of dating and relationships: being less focused on the outcome and enjoying the process, not taking yourself too seriously (always an attractive trait), and staying plucky in the face of possible rejection. Be clear on what you do and don't want and pack a burping cloth just in case.

MAGNETISM

Your vibe attracts your vibe. And we all want our vibe to be a reflection of our best self. It's an outward expression of your essence, which you identified in chapter 4, drawing people to your spirit. When two people's vibes generate attraction, it can be magnetic. The *law of attraction* suggests that what you decide you want from the universe will come to you. It's not magic; it's *manifesting*—a fun word to describe energy returning to you based on your efforts and attitude. In relationships, and especially in the world of dating, I suggest you manifest your magnetism to draw people who will appreciate you.

> There is a radiant splendor to your personality that has the capacity to draw and melt all hearts.
> —Shakti School

Magnetism is an example of nonverbal engagement. Flirting is another. Like sensuality and intimacy, *flirting* is a word that's been reduced to sex, even though all species engage in it for a variety of reasons. Let me reframe the word: flirting is a fun-loving, endearing, and sincere way to express yourself, connect, and be playful with someone else on your path forward—whether you're seeking a business deal or an amorous one. Flirting and being magnetic come more naturally to bodyful people because they're at ease in their body and aren't afraid to express their natural essence.

Adoring yourself, quirks and all, is magnetic. Self-adoration doesn't mean you think you're perfect in the Western sense of the word, as I described in chapter 5. It means that you are uniquely, perfectly *you* and find it pretty cool much of the time. As the poet Maya Angelou said, "I don't trust people who don't love themselves and tell me, 'I love you.' There is an African saying which is: Be careful when a naked person offers you a shirt."

CHEMISTRY

Magnetism is the heat that draws people together and chemistry is the spark. You can't plan or replicate chemistry, which is why it's so mystifying. If I could bottle that X factor I'd be a wealthy woman. You know it when you feel it—in your viscera, gut instinct, and subtle body energy—platonically or erotically. Either music is made together or it's not.

Obviously, things such as bad breath, body odor, distractibility (put those phones away), and being insecure can thwart chemistry. Behaviors such as eye contact, openness, and overlap in hobbies and values can maintain it. It's also powerfully biochemical. How someone smells—their pheromones—triggers animal instincts and the excitatory chemical dopamine. We can be junkies for that pleasure high, mistakenly equating it with longer-term states of happiness. Add oxytocin, the bonding hormone elicited during touch, and this is why new-relationship energy can be addictive. Those boosts of energy are an invitation to grow and expand your heart. I say ride that high! Just try to do so with bodyful awareness.

REUNION GRIEF

Sometimes the very thing your heart desires, such as a fulfilling partner, can initially provoke your deepest sorrow. Having your dream actually become a reality might shake up and release sadness for all those years you endured the longing. The relationship therapist Pat Love calls this *reunion grief*.[6] She compares it to a child who was away from his parents all week at camp. When they arrive to pick him up, he might be flooded with emotion and cry in their arms. What happened? Shouldn't he be happy to see them? His body has been holding on to pining for his parents all week and now it's safe to let out emotions because they are a container to soothe him. This can happen to adults when healthy love finally comes into their lives.

Reunion grief is an example of how the human body can suppress its desires for companionship for long periods of time. But once the heart's long-awaited cravings are met, stuffed emotions can gush out. If you're overcome with reunion grief, welcome what wants to move through your body. With time, you'll feel more stable to trust and welcome the pleasures of this new relationship.

There have always been complexities and contradictions within relationships that impact our personal and shared pleasures. The myths and distinctions I've pointed out are to question the assumptions and patterns we can fall into. It doesn't mean we have all the answers. It means we recognize the paradox, ambiguity, and potential within relationships. From there we can choose our connections more soulfully, which is at the core of living a bodyful life.

Erotic Pleasure

> This is one reason why the erotic is so feared, and so often relegated to the bedroom alone, when it is recognized at all. For once we begin to feel deeply all the aspects of our lives, we begin to demand from ourselves and from our life-pursuits that they feel in accordance with that joy which we know ourselves to be capable of.
>
> —*Audre Lorde*

WHETHER YOU'RE DABBLING in the dating world or celebrating decades with your beloved, the power and pleasure of erotic energy is possible for all. Erotic energy can be awakened by the different aspects of body intelligence that you've been cultivating. In hierarchical fashion, erotic and sexual pleasure blossom from all three layers of bodyfulness: from listening to your body's yearnings, limits, heartache, and hope; from knowing how to *engage* your body in ways you need; and from feeling unfettered and entitled to that pleasure zone with someone else.

There are so many transactional aspects to sex and eroticism—and I'm not talking here about a financial one. Sex and eroticism are an exchange of expectations, trust, emotions, support, an offering and receiving, a means of escape, a way to feel we matter, and beyond. It's a delicate balance. The sultry spiciness of eroticism may be hard to measure, but research on the benefits of pleasurable sex show that it's quite the elixir. Sexual satisfaction is linked to greater relationship satisfaction (no surprise there), authenticity, connection, being fully present, transcendence, deep intimacy, more exploration and risk, better communication, and vulnerability.[1] Other research has correlated sexual satisfaction with overall life satisfaction, mental and physical health, and happiness.[2] Women with more active and satisfying sexual relationships report higher ratings of overall emotional and relationship satisfaction (again, no surprise).[3] Seems too good to be true. But just ask the well-fucked people of the world and you can probably see it on their faces!

Erotic fireworks or not, a little sexual bonding goes a long way in connecting a relationship. I've found that when clients report their sex life as at least mediocre—happening from time to time and pleasant enough—it's *one* element of their relationship satisfaction. It might be lackluster at times or not happening as frequently as one or both would like, but it's good enough. But when the couple's sex life is nonexistent—as in no pulse—it can be a relationship deal breaker (certainly for the person who wants sex more). It's like hydration on a hike: If you bring your water bottle, you'll sip on it from time to time and not think much of it. But if you forget your water bottle, you might spend the whole hike noticing how parched you are and barely enjoy the view. The difference between having your sexual needs met just *a little* versus not at all is vast. I'm talking Grand Canyon.

Erotic pleasure relies on being at home in your body, present and awake, safe, and peaceful. It requires you to surrender to your sensations, breath, muscles, and body boundaries. If you let your mind wander or cling to control the whole time, you're not really *in* the experience. Some of this is cultural—if you spend twenty-three hours of your day trying to be in control, of course you'll struggle with relinquishing it when pleasure beckons you to be easy like Sunday morning. The bodyful tips I include at the end of the chapter can help you surrender that grip.

DESIRE DIFFERENCES

Imagine a match being struck along a matchbook in slow motion, building friction and heat, igniting a spark that turns into a hot flame. It has the power to light up the room. Once it's burned out, smoke fades into the ether. Just like that flickering flame, your sexual energy is not a constant. Desire's comings and goings—what lights it, keeps it lit, and what blows it out—ebb and flow throughout life and the course of a relationship.

Often I hear clients blame themselves for thinking they have a libido that's too high or too low. There's nothing wrong with their desire levels; syncing them with someone else's is just plain tricky. It could be due to any of these libido killers: growing distance, hectic work or kid schedules, falling out of love or like, fatigue, stress, hormones, injury, depression, lack of sleep, anxiety (including performance anxiety), being too self-conscious, having a guilty conscious, discomfort with sober sex, past trauma, questioning one's sexuality, or a major life event such as a death or newborn baby. Is your head spinning? Well, that interferes with erotic alchemy also.

If the low-desire person is not curious about *why* they feel that way, if they'd rather not deal with it or they make up excuses, they're probably stuck in shame or have an avoidant style, overregulating themselves with their arousal brakes on. The low-desire person has the control in the relationship, which is sometimes why they take that stance to begin with—they gotta dig their heels in somewhere. This leaves the other person hanging in the dark, wondering why they're being rejected.

The sex educator and author Emily Nagoski describes people as having two different arousal states.[4] When you're revved up, your "accelerator" is on. When you're not, your "brakes" are on. People who are in fight-flight-freeze mode of their nervous system typically have the brakes on. People in a rest-and-digest mode are calmer and therefore better able to feel their sexual energy—their accelerator is on. Nagoski explains that the accelerator starts differently for people: Some have *spontaneous desire*; they're able to get turned on more randomly, independent of obvious external cues. Others have *responsive desire*, which requires some coaxing to get their accelerator warmed up. Whichever camp you fall into, don't play the blame game. Understand that arousal styles vary, plan accordingly, and don't always take things too personally.

Pay attention to what generates excitement for you in general, not just erotically. Maybe it's the sound of someone's voice, the smell of cologne, or an old song. Now notice the opposite, what shuts you down. It could be the sound of kids arguing, a blustery wind, or the smell of something moldy. This is an invitation to go through each of the senses and recall what aroused you erotically in the past—even if it's been a minute.

Pleasure from sex might not be important to your relationship. For people who are asexual, it's not important at all. Someone can also *say* that sex is not important to them but they actually have deep-seated repression or trauma that interferes with their intimacy in ways they haven't faced. For others, sex can be a big part of their identity and what they value in a relationship.

A love life does not always mean an erotic life. This headline from the satirical newspaper *The Onion* jokingly captures that well: "Couple Spices Up Love Life by Adding Sex into Relationship." If you aren't interested in pleasure from sex, it doesn't mean there's something *wrong* with you, it means there is something blocking your erotic energy. Besides the people who are happily asexual, there are also people in the process of working through sexual trauma or pain during intercourse or focused on other life passions and pleasures, which is how life goes.

Navigate the differences by embracing nonsexual erotic pleasures. It could be touch—hugging, back rubs, cuddling, holding hands—or things such as stretching and exercising together; deep philosophical, intellectual, or emotional conversations that are stimulating; or being alongside each other in nature or enjoying art together. The pleasures of intimacy can come in many forms, and companionate love is also powerfully pleasurable and fulfilling.

MAINTAINING DESIRE

Pleasure is plentiful when a relationship is new and sparkly. But settling into a long-term relationship shatters the grand illusion of infatuation. As your chosen person sinks off the pedestal you put them on, you're at eye level with someone trying to figure out life just like you. Falling in lust, and then perhaps love if you're lucky,

> There is no settling down without a settling for.
> —Dan Savage

is the easy part. Still adoring each other through the carpool schedules and in-law visits is another matter. And when a couple has kids, their pleasures can get pushed aside as parenting becomes the priority. How do we preserve passion after sharing in the traffic jams and stomach flus of life?

As I mentioned in the last chapter on sexual intelligence, sex and our bodies are *supposed* to change over time. So too with desire. Part of erotic intelligence is not expecting things to stay the same as when you first met. Inevitably, something happens that the psychologist Jack Morin calls the "love/lust" split.[5] As the intimacy (oxytocin, trust, attachment) is dialed up, the sexual desire (dopamine, adrenaline, novelty) dials down. Next thing you know, monogamy can feel like monotony.

This is when sex transforms into sweatshirt sex, leftover sex, and sexorexia (not having any sex at all). With sweatshirt sex you're certainly not putting on lingerie, much less taking your sweatshirt off. You're not bothering with foreplay, because it's a miracle you're even being physical at all. The mystery may be gone, but it doesn't mean the tenderness is. Leftover sex, as coined by the sex therapist David Schnarch, is what you won't do and what they won't do, so you settle for what's leftover.

Let's face it—everyday life isn't simple or sexy (I suppose unless you and your partner embrace tantric philosophy, which sees the pleasure in even humdrum aspects of life). For most people, the higher their stress level, the lower their libido, which can also lower compassion and gratitude for a partner. No wonder people bump heads more once they're not "bumpin uglies," to quote '90s slang.

No matter what, every relationship evolves—some toward depth, some toward distance, and some a vacillation of the two. The thing is, you have to *cultivate* desire, it doesn't just show up like a genie in a bottle. So here are some bodyful suggestions to help give the relationship renewed vigor.

Like Your Body, Like Your Partner

If you don't want to be naked because you don't like your changing or aging body, no amount of lingerie or rabbit vibrators will change that. If this is you, explore the reasons why: Are you able to feel raw or vulnerable in other areas of your life? Do you allow yourself to *ever* feel pleasure? As I mentioned earlier in the book, assign yourself healthy pleasures in small doses. Exercise, meditation, music, artwork, cooking, and being outdoors are just some ways to engage your erotic self.

Even if you *like* your body well enough but you aren't connected to its emotional cues, you'll have less erotic desire. And even worse, research shows you could have more animosity toward your partner. One couple I worked with, Harry and Lola, had a level of tension in session that I could cut with a knife. Lola was always mad at Harry for something. I searched high and low for her reasons but it appeared Harry was a solid partner—patient, emotionally intelligent, and attentive to Lola. She was certainly not the first client who wanted me to "fix" their partner because everything was the other person's fault. I realized that Lola had some lifelong anger and control issues bottled up inside of her but was too disconnected from her body to do anything about it. So Harry became the easy target. Helping Lola become more bodyful meant she was able to recognize her emotions and take ownership for her reactivity. She learned ways to regulate that didn't involve Harry as her punching bag. Eventually their interactions became kinder and more enjoyable.

Body Gratitude

Have a daily practice of gratitude for your body. Gratitude is heart-full energy, guiding your nervous system and neural pathways to a moment of peace. Expand it to your partner as well: their spirit, sense of humor, that they emptied the litter box or cleaned the fridge—anything else big or small. What matters is that you're cultivating grateful feelings for them, a foreplay all its own. More frequent expressions of gratitude increase couples' sexual satisfaction by improving their emotional connection.[6]

Sensual Versus Savage

Sensuality is often used interchangeably with sexuality, but as we learned in chapter 10, it's a treasure chest all its own. Sensuality and sexuality are like wine and cheese; depending on the pairing, your taste buds can come alive as they enhance each other.

There can be many ways to embody pleasure through sex, with slow sensual touch on one end and rushed, getting-off sex on the other (what I called McDonald's sex in chapter 12). When sex is slow, tender, and savored, it can be sensually pleasurable. The space might include candles, music, comfy textures, and soft touch such as caressing and kissing. The alternative is faster, more aggressive, and the conditions of the space might not even matter. There's nothing inherently wrong with a quickie—more power to you in these busy times. Do what you gotta do to add variety or clean out your pipes; just make sure you aren't skipping over your senses every time. When you approach sex sensually, from a place of bodyfulness, you can experience a subtler, *slow-building pleasure*. If you're racing to a finish line every time, there are all sorts of delicious things you could miss along the way.

No matter the context, slowing down and taking the time to be present with someone is treasurable. Here are some sensual practices to include in the foreplay of your life.

Make your bed a sensual haven. Get the softest sheets, the fluffiest comforter, and pillows made of the right texture for you, and regularly update your mattress. You're supposed to be spending a third of your life there, sleeping or erotically playing, so don't let it get saggy and full of dust, for crying out loud. The bigger the bed the better, like an adult playpen to romp around in. Contrary to some people's belief that a bigger bed means you'll be less inclined to cuddle, bodyfulness can make you want to cuddle naturally, not just because you're confined by lack of space. Small beds make for cramped sleep and grumpy moods.

Engage in breast massage. For female bodies, let go of concerns about your breast size and invite your partner to massage them, kiss them, and pay attention to them. Not just a quick brushing over but lusciously engaging them with oils and different types of touch. Refer to the Chakra Four practices listed in the appendix to enhance this idea.

Increase eye contact. Eye contact is powerful. Science tells us that our eyes inform our nervous system and are the main channel to discern novelty. Eye gazing is a deeply intimate process, which might be a bit much for some. In which case, start by holding eye contact a little longer than you would normally, either in the bedroom or as you share a meal together. Notice the difference between eye-to-eye contact in front of each other and being side by side. Or you can do just the opposite: get all *Fifty Shades of Grey* and take turns being blindfolded.

Disagree? Let It Flow to Let It Go

Unresolved bickering doesn't inspire eroticism. But what if you went about it more bodyfully? Often couples argue while sitting across the table (or bed) from each other. Their hearts are pounding, blood vessels ready to pop, tension building . . . so take that show on the road. Get up and get moving. Process your disagreement on a walk, allowing your body's natural release and recalibration process to prevent a cold war. Can't leave the house? Leave the room separately instead. I don't care if you do push-ups, sun salutations, jumping jacks, or bucking like a bronco to get your agitation out. Then return to your partner later. This gives you both a chance to simmer down and transition from your reactive mind to a calmer mind.

Transgression

I once saw a magazine advertisement with the tagline "Just the right amount of wrong." There is excitement in transgression. It feels good to be "bad" because taking risks evokes dopamine. We often crave the most what we can't have. If you and your partner are committed to a monogamous relationship, you'll need to find ways to enliven your body from new and naughty activities, not other people. Even novel conversations create arousal. Professor Paul Bloom, the author of *How Pleasure Works*, explains that pleasure often comes from things that are new.[7] Partners doing novel activities together boost the brain's reward system. Rather than doing the same things over and over again (being too habituated), novelty helps you feel bonded as you both embrace and experience the unknown. Build and invest in something together, whether it be a cottage in the woods or taking your first picnic in years.

Space

Recently I heard the most requested thing celebrities ask for in real estate is having two master bedrooms. We all don't have that kind of disposable income, but the toll of feeling smothered may cost the relationship. As the saying goes, familiarity breeds contempt. There has been a movement over the past decade called *living apart together* (LAT). People in long-term relationships (even those that are married) are finding that separate residences help them look forward to seeing each other. Remove the unsexy tasks of domesticity and erotic energy builds in its absence.

Erotic Polarity

We may see couples who look and dress alike, but typically they didn't start off that way. They met as two people intrigued about someone *unlike* them. Erotic energy increases if people have different levels of masculine and feminine energy. The less alike you are, the more sexual tension; the more similar you are, the easier day-to-day life might be but the less erotic attraction. Oh, the paradox of it all. Complete the "Receptive and Projective Energy Exercise" (see appendix) to see where you land and then compare your results with your partner. It may remind you of the energetic differences that originally drew you to each other.

Erotic Blueprint

Most people have heard of the five love languages, which include acts of service, words, touch, gifts, and quality time.[8] But did you know there are five erotic languages? They include sensual, energetic, sexual, kink, and shape-shifter. This is the work of the sexual health coach Miss Jaiya, who has an Erotic Blueprint Breakthrough quiz to measure where your preferences land.[9] Knowing these similarities and differences prevents confusion or hurt feelings. Similar to the dosha constitution from chapter 9, when you learn how someone is hardwired, you're less likely to over-personalize their behavior.

Moving Meditations

One of the main influences of bodyfulness is yoga asana (poses), which have been shown to help people be more present, flexible, and have better breath control and regulation—all elements that optimize physical intimacy. The author Naomi Wolf found this to be the case: "Based on my research, the anecdotal evidence is that women who are happiest with their sex lives tend to do some sort of mind-body practice like yoga. Women who practice yoga may have more sensation because yoga supports spine health, which in turn supports circulation and engorgement."[10] Research has shown that practicing yoga regularly increases pelvic and abdominal muscle tone.[11] The physicality of breathing and moving alongside your babe—whether it be on the mat, the court, the field, or the pool—is direct practice for moving and breathing together erotically.

Healing Touch

My client Frank told me, "I just want someone to hold." He was a man in his late fifties who had been single for decades. The real issue was his social anxiety; he was a lifelong loner. As a result, he had a very small circle of friends. The only touch he received as a child was a spanking or hand slap, certainly not nurturing touch. Through our years working together he slowly left his comfort zone and joined meditation classes, started volunteering at an animal shelter, and began jamming guitars with a coworker. But he still didn't have shared touch in a loving way. I suggested he look into "cuddle parties" but this was understandably too anxiety provoking for him. So instead, he solicited cuddling a few times a year when his body begged for an embrace.

We all need loving touch to bond and reassure each other, to contain and calm our stress response. The hormone oxytocin is usually associated with mom-and-baby bonding while nursing, but it actually emerges from *any* human touch that we find pleasurable, even our own self-massage. Oxytocin increases attachment with someone and, even better, altruism in general.

The healing power of touch is why some people might be more verbally expressive after sex or cry after sex (not from physical pain). They're being deeply tended to. The words or tears are the body's way of releasing the past now that they're safe with someone they trust. Nestling with someone in a time of need can be all it takes to feel that everything's going to be alright. And relationships can be sustained in a really tender way by different expressions of touch when sex itself is not as available. It's medicine for our sense of separateness.

Sync Your Foreplay

One person's penchant for dirty talk can be another person's repulsion. My client Brenda wanted attention from her husband that felt sweet and romantic; it's what put her in the mood. His method—walking by and slapping her ass while she cooked—had quite the opposite effect. This left her feeling objectified, like she married a drunk frat boy. No wonder she had lost interest. Brenda would have sex with him out of obligation, much of the time gritting her teeth until the end. This was a violation her body absorbed time and time again; no wonder she began to dissociate from her body during sex and felt lonely in the relationship. It wasn't that her desire jumped ship but that she didn't desire the ways he offered it. We worked on her communication and things began to improve. You might not always be able to sync your friskiness, but you can share your preferences and shift things accordingly.

The organization OMGYes is dedicated to exploring ways to increase women's pleasure, and they have an instructional website with helpful videos. One of their many takeaways is that consistency of touch is important while approaching heightened excitement, but in the earlier build-up phase, variation of touch really heats things up (such as various paces, adding surprises, and orbiting *around* erogenous zones in a teasing way). For most women, foreplay is not to be overlooked; it's where erotic energy magnifies!

Kiss More and Talk Less

I'm not a fan of lots of talking *during* sex. Sure, it's important to express your edge, but too much talking pulls you out of your felt-sense experience and into a different hemisphere of your brain (less so if it's metaphorical language). If you feel the need to use your mouth, then kiss more, activating all those heightened nerve endings on your lips. Spend the first several minutes of physical intimacy only kissing, rather than rushing to the next pleasure point.

Sensual Communication Exercise

Have the lighting in the room high enough to see each other's eyes and facial expressions but not too bright; candles are helpful. Then decide who will be touched first and invite them to close their eyes. When you are the person doing the touching, start at your lover's feet and work your way up their body by using light, medium, and hard touch in different areas. When you are on the receiving end, avoid criticism of the person touching you, but do give them messages—yes or no, more or less, lighter or harder. When you are receiving touch, focus on the sensual feeling in your body and what the variations of touch elicit.

Review the Pleasure-Measure and Bodyfulness quizzes. You may have completed these earlier to get a baseline measure. If so, now it's time to take the quizzes again to see if your relationships with your body and with pleasure have evolved.

UNAPOLOGETIC PLEASURE

Another funny, but sadly true headline from *The Onion* read "Kinky Girlfriend Wants to Try Sexual Pleasure Tonight." As I shared in the first part of the book, women's sexual pleasure hasn't just been forgotten, there's been systematic backlash against it. Patriarchy fears a woman loving her curves who takes up space in the world. A sexually evolved woman was once considered a psychiatric illness by the medical field, but we've come a long way and now just consider her damaged and slutty. Sigh. I can feel my nervous system amp up in anger just typing that. Even things such as "women's intuition" have been mocked. And yet research shows women thirst for the frisson of a tryst just as much, if not more, than men do. Perhaps because research shows women get bored by sex earlier in the relationship compared to men.[12] Maybe *that's* the real reason why 38 percent of women report decreased or no desire for sex with their partner.[13]

> I finally know the difference between pleasing and loving, obeying and respecting. It has taken me so many years to be okay with being different, and with being this alive, this intense.
>
> —*Eve Ensler*

I hope this book helps end the legacy of disapproval for a woman who listens to her body's desires and proceeds with swagger to get them met, free from shame. My mentioning of my own "field research" in chapter 13 may have incited judgment from some. So be it, that's part of my job. What matters to me is that anyone who's been sexually marginalized embodies their sexual rights and desires unapologetically. It takes time and lived experience to understand what that means for you and to make intentional erotic choices.

No matter your age or where you fall on the gender spectrum, seeking hookups in a sideways attempt to feel better about yourself, or clinging to someone's approval of your body, gives literal meaning to the phrase "chasing tail." You will not catch the validation you're seeking. You can have total sexual freedom and satisfaction and still be unhappy. This is because the act of sex cannot fill an emptiness within your heart. Acting on your desires needs to come from a conscious place of radical self-love.

Start by being curious about your sexual motives. Think back to past intimate encounters and ask yourself, "What did I want from that exchange—moments of pleasure? A release of pent-up energy? To feel wanted? To feel sexy? To feel younger? To share myself with someone I care about?" Ideally your choices emanate from owning the desires you know you're entitled to, and from a place of fullness within yourself, not a reactive neediness for others to confirm you.

Beyond erotic pleasures, even a woman owning her desire for the pleasure of world travel or starting her own business can incite envy. I say this as a cautionary tale. There may be people who will feel threatened by you and throw shade your way. And it is not your job to shrink or apologize to them for the insecurities they feel. It is your job to keep shining your light and feeling your joy, whether it be a swim in a cold lake on a hot day or a friendly encounter with your neighbor on an airplane. Keep owning your right to pleasure and express it in the world. As you expand your pleasure potential, hopefully others model from you. Because you have goddess energy within you that wants to be expressed. As the writer Audre Lorde said, awareness and reverie for your body, and pleasures found in eroticism have powerful energies all their own: "The erotic is a resource within each of us that lies in a deeply female and spiritual plane, firmly rooted in the power of our unexpressed or unrecognized feelings. As women, we have come to distrust that power which rises from our deepest and non-rational knowledge."[14] Whole-body trust for your inner knowing and erotic powers flourishes as you bask in this third stage of bodyfulness. Support this intangible, ephemeral erotic power that you possess throughout your life span.

This book invited you to challenge the systems that say your mind is superior, that only certain bodies are superior, and that only certain relationships are superior. It has invited you to prioritize your pleasures in a healthy way and share them with others in the face of repression, shame, and limited access. It has invited you to listen to your body's primal needs and wants, not what the system tells you they should be. Channel your inner rebel and break free; reclaim the sovereignty of your body.

Bodyfulness reconnects you to your whole body by inhabiting your whole being, from your unique longings and appetites to the collective pulse of the earth's rhythms. Our history may have denied or misused the potential of our body, and the potential of pleasure, casting aside this aspect of human potential. It may have feared what is essentially the opposite of depression, anxiety, and separateness. But your body has patiently known all along what whole-person health feels like and whole-culture health looks like. And we are living proof that healing is possible. Your body has always known that pleasure is an emergent healing medicine, yours for the taking, waiting to be ignited. As you learn how to live in your body, you will recognize this with fresh eyes. As you listen to the voice of your heart, it will tell you what you need next.

What's on the other side of this revolution brewing within body-based medicine, this increasing acceptance of holistic practices, and the social movements demanding collective care of *all bodies* as sacred? I dream it's a place where every body has access and opportunity to healthy pleasures as a vibrant life-force energy and a generator of human-to-human intimacy. This is how we will transform a bodiless culture—one bodyful person at a time, one bodyful act at a time.

Appendix

THE PLEASURE-MEASURE QUIZ

The sixteen statements below offer a chance to measure your relationship to pleasure. For each statement, score your response using the 5-point scale below. Then add the four subtotals together to find your total score and corresponding pleasure-measure summary. Use this summary as a guide to the various ways you can enhance or shift your attitudes and behaviors toward pleasure for yourself, your body, and your relationships.

0	1	2	3	4	5
none of the time		some of the time		all of the time	

Sensual Pleasure

1. I am connected to my senses (smell, taste, sound, touch, sight). ____
2. I feel centered and present. ____
3. I take time to pause and feel gratitude. ____
4. I spend time in nature and the outdoors. ____

Subtotal: _____

Playful Pleasure

1. I engage in one or more hobbies in my life. ____
2. I find ways to connect to humor/laughter. ____
3. I engage in at least one activity that is not goal- or outcome-oriented. ____
4. I take time to be creative. ____

Subtotal: _____

Lively Pleasure

1. I have physical activities I become absorbed in. ____
2. I seek out opportunities for growth in my profession. ____
3. I like to travel to new places. ____
4. I have one or more activities where my focus becomes immersed. ____

Subtotal: _____

Erotic and Sexual Pleasure

1. I lack guilt or shame about my sexual thoughts, feelings, or behaviors. ____
2. I am aware of my sexual desires. ____
3. I talk openly about sexual health with people I trust when appropriate. ____
4. I seek physical intimacy in my romantic relationships. ____

Subtotal: _____

Personal Notes and Reflections:

Overall Total: _____

Date: _____

Scoring

0–40: *Dimly Lit* You struggle with staying connected to your body and being in the present moment. It's hard for you to give yourself moments of pleasure because you may get stuck in guilt, shame, perfectionism, overachieving, feeling the need to always be busy, taking care of others over yourself, struggling with attention and focus, or being caught in addiction (whether it be a person, substance, or other distraction method). For you, it's important to take baby steps: start by setting the intention to pause a couple of times a day to slow down, get centered, and ask, "What

do I really need right now? What does my body need right now?"
Connect more to your senses by introducing essential oils, clothing with soothing textures, and spending time in nature; add more
creativity and playfulness into your life, even if it's introducing a
little flare in how you dress or the way you decorate your space;
and begin to involve yourself in simple little pleasures scattered
throughout your week, with the mantra *I deserve this.*

41–60: *Flickering* You make the intention to have different types
of presence, play, and pleasure in your life in a balanced way—
which is awesome—although you might struggle with manifesting
it (due to barriers in the modern world or your own mental barriers) at times. Look at what might be getting in the way of having
more pleasure in your life: Is it hard for you to prioritize pleasure?
Is there something else you need to say no to in order to create
the space? Are there old messages from your upbringing that consciously or unconsciously interfere with you living out what is your
birthright of pleasure? Look at the places, people, and activities
that regulate you (either they light you up or simmer you down,
depending on what you need in the moment) and continue to prioritize them as important tools in your pleasure toolbox.

61–80: *On Fire, Baby!* You own your right to pleasure whether
it be sensual, playful, liveliness, or erotic/sexual, and no one can
take this away from you! You embody these concepts as regular practices in your life, even when things get busy. You've got
a great foundation of connecting to your senses, presence, and
ease; bringing in humor, creativity, and playfulness; finding flow
and immersing in work or leisure activities; and being sexually
and erotically liberated. However, notice if all this pleasuring
prevents you from coping with discomfort, frustration, or the
necessary hard work that's required at times. For people in this
score range finding balance is key, and it's important to practice
tolerating the less pleasurable aspects of life with some patience,
teeth-gritting hard work, or the art of surrendering.

RECEPTIVE AND PROJECTIVE
ENERGY EXERCISE

The principle of yin and yang is about all things existing as contradictory opposites in nature. Sun and moon. Day and night. Inhale and exhale. The holistic health advocate Deepak Chopra said, "These apparent opposites have real effects on your lives. You think, behave, and feel according to the cultural expectations and norms that are held around these binaries."[1] This includes the binary of male and female, which I refer to here as projective and receptive energies, respectively.

For this exercise, try to let go of your beliefs about men versus women as genders and think in terms of different types of energy that *all* humans have within them. Let this exercise shine light on different aspects of yourself to help you become aware of what you value and any imbalances you have. Although the main point of this exercise is to recognize and encourage the side that is underdeveloped, it could also help you notice what you're drawn to in relationships (the idea that opposites attract, and two people are complementary in their differences). Of course, although *attraction* is based on opposite or complementary energy, the fabric of long-lasting emotional intimacy requires more than merely attraction, as I discussed in part three.

Circle the words in the column that most apply to you and count the totals at the bottom.

Receptive Energy	Projective Energy
Intuitive	Present
Grounded	Nonjudgmental
Receptive	Disciplined
Reflective	Focused

Receptive Energy	Projective Energy
Supportive	Logical
Vulnerable	Confident
Authentic	Protective
Empathetic	Honest
Open	Accountable
Trusting	Integrity
Creative	Holds boundaries
Compassionate	Responsible
Nurturing	Assertive

Totals: _____

Out of balance, this energy looks like:

Receptive Energy	Projective Energy
Insecure	Controlling
Needy	Aggressive
Manipulative	Competitive
Inauthentic	Unstable
Overly emotional	Confrontational
Victim	Wants power

Totals: _____

BODY CONVERSATION

This Body Conversation exercise encourages you to cultivate a curious mind toward your body. It's a guide to help you practice tuning in to the currents and impulses that flow through your body and to help you be more aware of your physical, emotional, and energetic body. Refer to this repeatedly to help cultivate embodied mindfulness.

What am I generally noticing in my body right now:

My right side feels:

My left side feels:

The front of my body feels:

The back of my body feels:

Within my body feels:

My overall breathing pattern feels:

My inhale feels:

My exhale feels:

My overall sensations feel:

Smell:

Sound:

Touch:

Taste:

Sight:

My stomach and abdomen feel:

    If they were a color(s) they would be:

    What is my digestion telling me today?

Where could I soften in my body?

What might want acknowledgment in my body?

    of pain/discomfort/fatigue:

    of ease/peace/steadiness:

    of strength/empowerment/confidence:

    of stagnation/cobweb feeling/stuckness:

If your body could do any movements right now (not caring how it looks to others), what would they be? Pick three and do them now.

If your voice could make any sounds right now (not caring how it sounds to others), what would they be? Pick three and make them now. If it feels weird, wait until you're by yourself.

BODYFULNESS QUIZ

The twelve statements below offer a chance to measure your relationship with your body as a resource for healing and joy. Once again, score each statement using the 5-point scale. The total score will correspond to the summaries on the next page that offer insight into your connection with your body and suggest ways to strengthen that connection—whether you scored 0 or 60.

0	1	2	3	4	5
none of the time		some of the time		all of the time	

1. I find aspects of my body to be strong. ____
2. I enjoy challenging my body physically. ____
3. I give my body what it needs for sleep and rest. ____
4. I notice and respond to my body when it is hungry and when it is full. ____
5. I listen to my body when it wants to socialize or be alone. ____
6. I like aspects of my body's appearance. ____
7. I trust my intuition and follow through with what it tells me. ____
8. I appreciate what my body does for me. ____
9. I allow myself to release with sound, whether it be crying, sighing, grunting, singing, etc. ____
10. I engage in massage or other types of therapeutic bodywork (acupuncture, yoga, tai chi, foam rolling, etc.). ____
11. I notice and connect with my breathing patterns. ____
12. I'm aware of what foods agree with me and eat accordingly. ____

Total: _____

Scoring

0–28: *Disembodied . . . Dissing Your Body* You tend to be immersed in thoughts, logic, rationality; you overthink things and aren't well connected to your body. Either you don't like your body because of pain or societal messages about how it "should be," or you simply ignore it and can't be bothered by it because you don't see the benefit. Your job is to start seeing how your body is a resource in your life: create a practice of moving your body and connecting to your breath each and every day, in a variety of ways, during which you become curious (rather than critical) about the language of your body and what it's telling you. Let it be experimental, a little investigating within yourself. Find daily gratitude in some aspect of your physical, emotional, and/or energetic body to acknowledge the subtle and not-so-subtle ways these different aspects are showing up for you. Your mantra is *My body is wise.*

29–45: *More Embodied* You try to have balance between your mind and your body and can discern what your body is asking for. You have some activities—whether it be movement and exercise or more therapeutic bodywork—that help you stay connected to your body. You generally listen to your energy levels and this informs whether you spend time by yourself or with others, which helps you stay centered. You try to trust your intuition but might not always follow through with what it's telling you. You might want to ramp up how often you pause and listen to your body's whisperings, and keep working to find delight and gratitude for what it's doing for you.

46–60: *Bodylicious* You are someone who resides in that beautiful body of yours. You listen to it and act accordingly, which helps you stay grounded, centered, and connected to your inner knowing on the one hand, and celebratory and sensual in your body on the other hand. You use your body as a resource to regulate yourself and feel good. Notice if there are times when you're operating too much out of emotionality or impulse and be sure to pause, step back, and take time to be alone. This can help you get perspective in order to bring some rationality or structure into the moment at hand.

LANGUAGE OF SENSATIONS

This table explains the sounds and behaviors the body makes when it's in the fight mode, flight mode, freeze mode, and at ease. Naturally, we all want to be in that fourth column as much as possible. As you become more conversant in the language of your sensations, hopefully you'll start to experience some of those sounds and peculiarities your body makes in a more welcoming way.

UNDER STRESS: FIGHT OR FLIGHT	UNDER STRESS: FREEZE OR DISSOCIATION	RELEASE/ DISCHARGE	SAFETY, EASE, PLEASURE, JOY, BLISS
Tight, constructed, contracted	Spacey, spaced out, zoned out	Tingling, tingly	Open
Bracing, braced	Foggy, fuzzy	Pulsing, pulsating	Steady
Tense, hard	Hard to focus (mind, vision, hearing)	Vibrating	Relaxed
Pain, painful	Sleepy, tired, no energy, drowsy	Radiating heat, hot, warm	Loose
Achey, aching	Light-headed	Chills, cooling down	Calm, still
Agitated	Dizzy	Trembling	Expansive
Restless	Swirling, spinning	Shaky, shaking	Spacious
Jittery, jumpy	Wobbly	Shivery, shivering	Grounded
Wound up	Dense	Quivery, quivering	Centered, aligned
Racing	Nauseous	Popping	Smooth

UNDER STRESS: FIGHT OR FLIGHT	UNDER STRESS: FREEZE OR DISSOCIATION	RELEASE/ DISCHARGE	SAFETY, EASE, PLEASURE, JOY, BLISS
Fluttering	Thick	Electric	Quiet
Clammy	Limp, flaccid muscles	Moving down, melting	Symmetrical
Pressure, pressured	Heavy	Water/sand moving down limbs	Soft
Jagged	Weighty, weighted down	Tears (crying or just teary)	Light
Dry mouth	Collapsed	Laughing	Bright
Heart beating fast, pounding	Sluggish, weak	Burping, gurgling in stomach	Fluid, flowing
Hard to breathe, shallow breath	Numb, empty, blank, hollow, flat	Yawning	Present
Holding breath	Blocked, stuck	Stretching	Alert
Jumble	Stiff	Bubbling, bubbly	Energized
Clenching, clenched	Frozen, paralyzed	Twitchy, twitching	Airy
On pins and needles	Not present	*See Note	Whole

Note: If any of the above sensations are always present, repetitive, and/or feel out of control and do not shift to sensations of relief, ease, and joy, it is not a release/discharge. Rather, it is a sign of misfiring in the nervous system in an attempt to release/discharge.

It should also be noted that the same expression may mean two completely different states. "Floating" may reflect a pleasant state or it could be a state of check-out and not centered.

—*Table influenced by the Somatic Experiencing® Trauma Institute*

AYURVEDIC DOSHA QUIZ

The chart below helps you to determine your doshic blueprint. Circle the qualities in the column that pertain to you. Keep in mind that many people have a primary dosha and a secondary dosha. For each characteristic, try to pick from one column, but you can circle from more than one if necessary. You will receive a total score that corresponds to a summary with specific lifestyle tips to reclaim balance.

CHARACTERISTICS	VATA (AIR)	PITTA (FIRE)	KAPHA (EARTH)
BODY FRAME	thinner for my build, flexible	medium for my build, muscular	bigger for my build, solid
WEIGHT	easy to lose, hard to gain	easy to lose, hard to gain	hard to lose, easy to gain
SKIN	cold to touch, dry	warm to touch, soft	cool to touch, oily
SWEAT	barely	profusely	moderately
HAIR	dry, coarse, curly	fine, straight, light	oily, thick, shiny
APPETITE	varies	intense	regular
DIGESTION	delicate, eat quickly	strong, can eat anything	eat and digest slowly
ELIMINATION	erratic or constipated	regular, loose	regular, slow
LEAST FAVORITE WEATHER	cold	hot	damp
BODY TEMP	hands and feet cold	warm	cool
SPEECH	talkative, may ramble	purposeful, direct	slow, cautious
EMOTION	fear	anger	confrontation avoidant

CHARACTERISTICS	VATA (AIR)	PITTA (FIRE)	KAPHA (EARTH)
MEMORY	learns quickly when not distracted, forgets easily	learns quickly, forgets slowly	requires more effort to learn, forgets slowly
ENERGY	wears out easily	can handle many activities	stamina, steady
ACTIVITY	always on the go	purposeful, competitive	prefers leisure activities
WALK	quickly	determinedly	slow and steady
SEX DRIVE	varies	intense	steady
CONFLICT MAKES ME . . .	anxious, restless	intense, irritable	lazy, depressed
MOOD	changes quickly	changes slowly	mostly steady
UNDER STRESS	easily excited	angry or critical	easygoing
LEARNING STYLE	short attention span	detail-oriented, good focus	"big picture" person, sustained focus
DECISION-MAKING	lots of ideas but changes mind	gathers lots of facts before making opinion	stubborn, makes up mind quickly
PROJECTS	strong start, hard to finish	organized, follows through	slow start, strong finish
FRIENDS	makes easily and changes often	work related	long-lasting
MONEY	shops often, spends	spends on special items	good at saving money, collects things
SLEEP	poor sleeper, fitful, can't recall dreams	good sleeper, often recalls dreams	sound, hard to wake up, recalls intense dreams
PERSONALITY	creative, imaginative	efficient, perfectionist	caring, patient

Totals

Vata: _____

Pitta: _____

Kapha: _____

Below are your results. If you have a constitution of more than one dosha, explore both to see what makes sense for you, factoring in how the seasons might impact them as well.

Mostly Vata

Air dosha: elements of space, air, and wind

Words to remember: grounding, warming, routine

Your air energy is increased by: windy, cool weather

In balance: joyful, free spirit, friendly, flexible, imaginative, easy breezy, active, creative, gifted with expression and communication

Out of balance: a hurricane, anxious, bodily disorders related to dryness and dehydration (constipation, skin irritations), spacey, insomnia, variable energy, and poor circulation

Tip: Start each day with something warm and packed with protein to ground you, rather than a jolt of caffeine as you head out the door. Implement one morning and evening ritual to help center you.

Mostly Pitta

Fire dosha: elements of fire and water

Words to remember: cooling, calming, moderation

Your fire energy is increased by: hot and sunny weather

In balance: joyful, sharp, courageous, driven, ease of laughter

Out of balance: too controlling, bossy, intense, fiery, volatile, overbearing, skin breaks out with acne or rashes, easily hangry (angry when hungry), heartburn

Tip: Find cooling foods, weather, and activities to temper you. Notice when you're getting overly competitive and try to let go and enjoy the process.

Mostly Kapha

Earth dosha: elements of water and earth

Words to remember: moving, stimulating, expression

Your earth energy is increased by: cold, wet weather

In balance: nourishing, loving, affectionate, calm, deep sleeper, regular appetite, team player

Out of balance: prone to depression, lethargy, sluggishness, weight gain, slow response, feeling easily hurt, heavy, dependent

Tip: Break from your routine and shake things up with novelty or adventure. Start each day with at least fifteen minutes of stretching to prevent stagnation.

CHAKRA EXERCISES

An over-reliance on the mind and limited focus on the body, including the energetic body, causes imbalances. Here are some suggestions to help you feel more balanced in your subtle body energy, chakra by chakra.

First Chakra: Root In

Theme: Earth—solid and dense, survival, basic needs, security, self-preservation, trust, raw feelings.
Area of the body: Feet, legs, pubic bone, first three vertebrae, bladder, colon, bones, and teeth.

When this chakra is balanced, you feel safe, grounded, and comfortable in your body; you have good immunity, an ability to relax, can maintain financial stability, and you're connected to nature. Fear blocks it.

Chakra 1 Practices

If you're in excess, try to let go of rigid boundaries, greed, and fear of change. Be generous by giving away a few things you like.

If you're blocked, you're functioning out of fear and don't feel safe. Connect to your body with lots of movement and touch, such as self-massage. Ground yourself by kneading your hands into the large muscle groups of your legs or use a foam roller. Notice your feet, the strength of your legs, and how your core strength helps balance you. Practice Child's pose.

Second Chakra: Motion Is Lotion

Theme: Accepting emotions and feelings; creativity, going with the flow, sweetness, sensuality, sexuality, and your right to pleasure. As you can probably guess, this chakra is my favorite—the seat of pleasure.
Area of the body: Low back, hips, genitals, lower abdomen. The hip joints (which includes the pelvis and thigh bones) are

the largest joints surrounded by the largest muscle tissues of the glutes, all near the organs of reproduction. Suffice it to say, this is quite an energy center of the body!

My main influence on the chakras comes from the chakra expert Anodea Judith, who explained that the first chakra lays the foundation for the second, like a cup of water: the first chakra is the cup, and the second chakra is the water. If your second chakra is overflowing (excessive), your cup runs over. You tend to be too emotional and need more boundaries. If your cup has run dry (deficient), you tend toward emotional numbness, rigidity, and fear of pleasure.[2]

Guilt blocks the second chakra and, as we've discussed, it certainly interferes with pleasure. While guilt in small doses can be a valuable source of feedback, when out of balance it blocks us and leads to all-or-nothing thinking. Balancing the second chakra involves reclaiming your right to *all* your feelings, even the ones you'd prefer not to have. When the energy of the second chakra is balanced and healthy, you are fluid, allowing yourself to feel and desire freely without guilt, understanding that you are entitled to it. You know how to find balance between your emotional and rational self.

Chakra 2 Practices

If you're blocked, connect with water: soak, float, steam, surf, tube, paddle board, or swim. Embrace what the somatic therapist Michaela Boehm describes as the more feminine energy of "flow mode"—softness and receptivity—rather than an aggressive "go mode." Accept and appreciate your emotions and feelings as valid sources of information. Do anything that gets you flowing: dance, pulse, sway, and find rhythm. If you're excessive, practice containment, exert stronger boundaries (say no), let go of being a people pleaser, and try to not over-identify with your feelings. Fortunately, much of this book is about maintaining a balanced second chakra, so keep staying the course.

For both excessive and blocked, strengthen your pelvic floor. It's important to maintain strength in the pelvic floor particularly as we age. In women, this "wonder of down under" is composed of the muscles, ligaments, connective tissues, and nerves that support the bladder, uterus, vagina, and rectum. In men (yes, men have a pelvic floor), it includes the muscles, tissues, and nerves that support the bladder, rectum, and other pelvic organs. The pelvic floor works in conjunction with other muscles of the inner core (including the diaphragm) to control pressure within the pelvis and abdomen to stabilize you. Whether it be continence or core stability, it behooves you to keep this area strong (as opposed to tense, which happens when there's been trauma to the area). Engage what yogis call your bandhas (core locks) by engaging and releasing the perineum and abdominal muscles to provide support, lift, and centering.

Third Chakra: Work It

Theme: Personal power, will, self-definition, confidence, responsibility, sense of humor.
Area of the body: The navel to the breastbone, called the *solar plexus*. This is your effort and your fire. It takes effort to get shit done! But it's more than just self-discipline; it's about balancing your drive with humor, playfulness, and warmth toward others. Shame blocks you here, causing you to question your worth.

Chakra 3 Practices

If you're blocked: Do vigorous activity, especially any core exercises such as forearm planks, sit-ups, or even standing on one leg and karate-kicking the other leg (bonus if you pair it with audible release such as a "ha!" sound). Find adventure to get out of your comfort zone and build self-confidence. If you're excessive: Curtail your need to be right. Try to let go of control. Find some things that are not goal-oriented (like everything I've mentioned in the section on playful pleasure in chapter 2).

These first three chakras are more about physicality. They're the base of your mountain. With an imbalanced first, second, and third chakra, I think of the quote by the author Geneen Roth: "Life becomes about your limitations, what you can and cannot do. How much you can hide. How ashamed you are of yourself. You close down your senses, you leave the world of sounds, of color, of laughter in favor of a reality you've created yourself."[3]

Fourth Chakra: Love Is Love

Theme: Love, connection, relationships, peace, altruism, compassion, gratitude.
Area of the body: Heart area, mid chest, sternum.

This is about loving others and receiving love. Self-acceptance and acceptance of others. It is blocked by grief, loss, and a lack of self-love.

Chakra 4 Practices

If you're blocked: Acknowledge yourself for something every day. Practice *metta* meditation, also known as loving-kindness meditation, to increase empathy. Let yourself cry. Ask yourself, "What's at the heart of this? What do I truly care about?" Practice heart openers in yoga, such as lying on your back and putting a bolster or pillow between your shoulder blades to lift and open the upper chest. If you're excessive: Try to let go of jealousy. Firm up your relationship boundaries. Remember, there are many sources of love in the world; it doesn't come solely from one person. If you're in a relationship, practice differentiation, which I mentioned in chapter 12.

For both excessive and blocked individuals, do a daily gratitude journal. And for women, give your breasts some love. Tantric philosophy sees the breasts, positioned at each side of the heart center, as "the guardians of the heart." It suggests you stimulate your breast tissue to tend to your heart, to experience pleasure, and to increase your ojas. I find this view—seeing your breasts as a source of your own pleasure rather than as solely for someone *else's* enjoyment (breastfeeding, male pleasure, or advertisements)—so refreshing.

Fifth Chakra: If You Want to Sing Out, Sing Out

Theme: communication (writing, dancing, verbal), self-expression, speaking your truth, good listener, creative, sense of timing and rhythm.

Area of the body: throat, neck, thyroid, parathyroid glands, jaw, mouth, and tongue.

Lies, mixed messages, secrets, and excessive criticism block this chakra.

Chakra 5 Practices

If you're blocked: Do more sighing and guttural sounds to release energy. Write in a journal. Practice using your voice to tell people about your dreams, your calling, your ideas. If you're excessive: Suggest they tell you this in return, so you can practice listening. Pause before you blurt something out, so you mean what you say and say what you mean. Practice more silent meditation.

Sixth Chakra: The Visionary

Theme: Intuition, perception, imagination, visualization, memory, dream recall.

Area of the body: Forehead, brow, between the eyebrows; referred to as the "third eye."

This is about knowing what you know; "seeing" in many different ways. Illusions block you. Growing up in a household in which what you saw was denied or did not match with what you were told, clouds your intuition.

Chakra 6 Practices

As the author and activist Toni Cade Bambara said, "The role of the artist is to make the revolution irresistible." We need imagination to build the future we all deserve. If you're blocked: Listen to your intuition and actually follow its warnings (all this body connection in the book should help). Take time to engage in fantasy, study mythology, or write down your dreams each morning. Rub your temples and brow with essential oils. Paint with watercolors for visual stimulation. Dress more colorfully.

If you're excessive: Stop obsessing or ruminating by coming back to your body. Associate images with feelings and physical outlets. If you have nightmares, be curious about the underlying message your subconscious is trying to tell you and work toward resolution.

Seventh Chakra: The Crown

Theme: Awareness, enlightenment, spiritual connection to your higher self, what's bigger than us, and the mystery of life.
Area of the body: Crown of the head, cerebral cortex.

This is about knowing, learning, spirituality, and open-mindedness. You become blocked if you're overly attached or fixated on external things or belief systems, or have a need to control the outcome.

Chakra 7 Practices

To find balance, you need to either face something emotionally *or* let something go (which also requires letting go at your third chakra, the ego). This is about realizing your true nature and letting go of petty concerns. Physically practice balance by having free-flowing movement, gazing at images such as a flame or mandala, or doing guided relaxations. To release excessive energy (overintellectualizing or spiritual addiction): do a scalp rub; legs up the wall for at least ten breaths; inhale your arms high above you and squeeze your fists at the top, then exhale your arms softly back down.

FLUID, NOT FLOODED EXERCISE

1. Put your feet firmly on the ground.
2. Feel all four corners of your feet on the earth and notice your stability.
3. Bend your knees if they're locked and bounce a few times with your knees and legs.
4. While keeping your legs in their same position, sway and twist your upper body from right to left, letting your arms dangle, feeling an opening in your spine.
5. Pause, look around your surroundings and name what colors and objects you see.
6. Bring your hands to your core and spread your fingers wide. Take five full belly breaths, feeling the rise and fall of your abdomen.
7. Relax your jaw, opening and closing it a few times.
8. Let out any guttural sounds such as a sigh, a moan, or an "ahhhh."
9. Shake your right hand, then your left hand, then both hands.
10. Shake your right foot, then your left foot, then alternate back and forth.
11. Shake your hands and your feet and your whole body.
12. Bring your feet wide, bend your knees, and fold forward to a "rag doll" position. Dangle your upper body for eight to ten breaths.

HEAD, HEART, GUT, GROIN MOVING MEDITATION

We all have different parts of ourselves and wear different hats. This exercise connects with four different parts of your physical and emotional self to help you integrate them. As you move through each area of your body, give attention to how it responds to the movements in the moment. Then reflect on what patterns tend to show up in that area of your body and how it might negate or encourage another area of your body. For example, does your head talk your heart out of being vulnerable? Does your gut inform your head on a decision? Be inquisitive about the interplay between these areas of your body.

Head

Start by rubbing your scalp with your fingers. After several breaths, move your hands down to your neck and upper shoulders, massaging these areas for several breaths.

Heart

Inhale as you extend your arms out wide, lifting your chest and arching your back slightly as you look up. Exhale and draw your arms back to the center of your chest, as if you're pulling the surrounding air to your heart, bringing one hand on top of the other. Repeat eight to ten times, expanding your chest with each inhale.

Gut

Move your hands to your stomach and take ten belly breaths, distending your lower abdomen. Think of your belly as a balloon getting filled up and released.

Groin

Stand up, bring your hands to your hips, and make big circles with your hips eight to ten times in one direction, then eight to ten times in the other direction. Keeping your hands on your hips, tilt your pelvis forward and back eight to ten times, as if you were doing Cat-Cow with your pelvis and frontal hip bone area.

Trauma Resource Guide

American Trauma Society. "Resources for Survivors." Trauma Survivors Network. Accessed December 7, 2020. https://www.trauma-survivorsnetwork.org/pages/resources-for-survivors.

Atkinson, Matt. *Letters to Survivors: Words of Comfort for Women Recovering from Rape*. Oklahoma City: RAR Books, 2011.

Burke Harris, Nadine. *The Deepest Well: Healing the Long-Term Effects of Childhood Adversity*. Boston: Mariner Books, 2018.

Emerson, David, and Elizabeth Hopper. *Overcoming Trauma Through Yoga: Reclaiming Your Body*. Berkeley, CA: North Atlantic Books, 2011.

Heller, Laurence, and Aline LaPierre. *Healing Developmental Trauma: How Early Trauma Affects Self-Regulation, Self-Image, and the Capacity for Relationship*. Berkeley, CA: North Atlantic Books, 2012.

Levine, Amir, and Rachel Heller. *Attached: The New Science of Adult Attachment and How It Can Help You Find—and Keep—Love*. New York: TarcherPerigee, 2010.

Levine, Peter A. *In an Unspoken Voice: How the Body Releases Trauma and Restores Goodness*. Berkeley, CA: North Atlantic Books, 2010.

Menakem, Resmaa. *My Grandmother's Hands: Racialized Trauma and the Pathway to Mending Our Hearts and Bodies*. Las Vegas: Central Recovery Press, 2017.

Myss, Caroline. *Anatomy of the Spirit: The Seven Stages of Power and Healing*. New York: Harmony, 2017.

van der Kolk, Bessel. *The Body Keeps the Score: Brain, Mind, and Body in the Healing of Trauma*. New York: Penguin, 2015.

van Dernoot Lipsky, Laura, and Connie Burk. *Trauma Stewardship: An Everyday Guide to Caring for Self While Caring for Others.* San Francisco: Berrett-Koehler Publishers, 2009.

Wolynn, Mark. *It Didn't Start with You: How Inherited Family Trauma Shapes Who We Are and How to End the Cycle.* New York: Penguin, 2017.

Notes

INTRODUCTION

1. Israel Shenker, "E.B. White, Notes and Comment by Author" *New York Times*, July 11, 1969, https://archive.nytimes.com/www.nytimes.com/books/97/08/03/lifetimes/white-notes.html.
2. Jalal Al Din Rumi, *The Essential Rumi* (New York: HarperCollins, 2010).

2. PLEASURE IS THE MEASURE

1. John Bradshaw, *Healing the Shame that Binds You*, rev.ed. (Deerfield Beach, FL: Health Communications, 2005).
2. Manuela Mischke-Reeds, *Somatic Psychotherapy Toolbox: 125 Worksheets and Exercises to Treat Trauma and Stress* (Eau Claire, WI: PESI Publishing, 2018), 105.
3. James Hillman, *The Myth of Analysis: Three Essays in Archetypal Psychology* (Chicago: Northwestern University Press, 1960), 48.
4. Steven Kotler, *The Rise of Superman: Decoding the Science of Ultimate Human Performance* (London: New Harvest, 2014).
5. Robert L. Maddex, "The Health Benefits of Sexual Expression," in *Encyclopedia of Sexual Behavior and the Law* (Washington, DC: CQ Press, 2006), 244–45.
6. Emily Bobrow, "What's Wrong with Infidelity?," *Economist*, November 22, 2016, https://www.economist.com/1843/2016/11/22/whats-wrong-with-infidelity.
7. Julie Peters, "The Soul Body Connection," *Spirituality and Health*, September/October, 2015.

3. EXPRESSION, NOT REPRESSION

1. David Ley, "Overcoming Religious Sexual Shame," *Psychology Today*, August 23, 2017, https://www.psychologytoday.com/us/blog/women-who-stray/201708/overcoming-religious-sexual-shame.
2. Morris Berman, *Coming to Our Senses: Body and Spirit in the Hidden History of the West* (Brattleboro, VT: Echo Point Books, 2015).
3. Christine Caldwell, *Bodyfulness: Somatic Practices for Presence, Empowerment, and Waking Up in Life* (Boulder: Shambhala, 2018), xxvii.

4. Graham Hart and Kaye Wellings, "Sexual Behaviour and Its Medicalisation: In Sickness and in Health," *British Medical Journal*, no. 324 (2002): 896–900, https://doi.org/10.1136/bmj.324.7342.896.

5. World Association for Sexual Health, "Sexual Health for the Millennium: A Declaration and Technical Document," (Minneapolis, MN: World Association for Sexual Health, 2008).

6. Michele Hutchison and Rina Mae Acosta, "They Raise the World's Happiest Children, So Is It Time You Went Dutch?" The *Telegraph*, January 7, 2017, https://www.telegraph.co.uk/family/parenting/raise-worlds-happiest-children-time-went-dutch/.

7. Cody C. Delistraty, "The Importance of Eating Together," The *Atlantic*, July 18, 2014, https://www.theatlantic.com/health/archive/2014/07/the-importance-of-eating-together/374256/.

8. Hutchison and Acosta, "World's Happiest Children."

9. Anthony Jackson, "Creativity in Schools: What Countries Do (Or Could Do)," Education Week (website), April 11, 2013, https://blogs.edweek.org/edweek/global_learning/2013/04/creativity_in_schools_what_countries_do_or_could_do.html.

10. Hear more from the Tara Brach podcast and from www.TaraBrach.com.

4. BOYS WILL BE BOYS

1. Sarah Right, "Today's Masculinity Is Stifling," The *Atlantic*, June 11, 2018, https://www.theatlantic.com/family/archive/2018/06/imagining-a-better-boyhood/562232/.

2. Elizabeth Sweet, "Beyond the Blue and Pink Toy Divide," TEDxUCDavis Talk, April 2015, 16:49, https://www.elizabethvsweet.com/tedx-talk.

3. Glennon Doyle, *Untamed*, (New York: Dial Press, 2020).

4. Ipek Ilkkaracan and Gulsah Seral, "Sexual Pleasure as a Woman's Human Right: Experiences from a Grassroots Training Program in Turkey," (Istanbul, Turkey: Women for Women's Human Rights, 2000), http://kadininin sanhaklari.org/wp-content/uploads/2018/06/SexualPleasure.pdf.

5. Bridget Christie, "Bridget Christie: A Joke about Plastic Surgery," April 22, 2020, in *Netflix Is a Daily Joke*, podcast, 4:59, https://netflix-is-a-daily-joke.simplecast.com/episodes/bridget-christie-a-joke-about-plastic-surgery-D3UZJ8YT.

6. Elaine Hatfield and Richard Rapson, *Love, Sex, and Intimacy: Their Psychology, Biology, and History* (New York: HarperCollins, 1993).

7. Peggy Orenstein, *Boys & Sex: Young Men on Hookups, Love, Porn, Consent, and Navigating the New Masculinity*, (New York: HarperCollins, 2020).

8. Peggy Orenstein, "Will We Ever Figure Out How to Talk to Boys About Sex?" *New York Times*, January 10, 2020, https://www.nytimes.com/2020/01/10/opinion/sunday/boys-sex.html.

9. Doug Braun-Harvey, "TU 42: Sexual Vitality, Refreshing Our Understanding of Sexual Health with Doug-Braun Harvey (Part 1 of 2)," June 28, 2018, in *Therapist Uncensored*, podcast, 52:10. https://www.youtube.com/watch?v=UbUlL7-h4_4.

10. Elizabeth Sully et al., "Adding It Up: Investing in Sexual and Reproductive Health 2019" (New York: Guttmacher Institute, 2020), https://www.guttmacher.org/report/adding-it-up-investing-in-sexual-reproductive-health-2019.

11. Orenstein, "Will We Ever Figure Out."

12. Orenstein, "Will We Ever Figure Out."

13. Elroy Boers, Mohammad H. Afzali, Patricia Conrod, "Temporal Associations of Screen Time and Anxiety Symptoms Among Adolescents," *The Canadian Journal of Psychiatry* 65, no. 3 (November 4, 2019): 206–8, https://doi.org/10.1177/0706743719885486.

14. Danielle Cohen, "Why Kids Need to Spend Time in Nature." Child Mind Institute (website), https://childmind.org/article/why-kids-need-to-spend-time-in-nature/.

5. NOT TONIGHT, HONEY, I'D RATHER INSTAGRAM

1. Paul Batalden, "Like Magic? ('Every system is perfectly designed . . .')," compiled by IHI Multimedia Team, Institute for Healthcare Improvement (website), August 21, 2015, http://www.ihi.org/communities/blogs/origin-of-every-system-is-perfectly-designed-quote.

2. Alberto Nardelli, "The French Take More Holidays and Work Less, but Does It Matter?" The *Guardian*, June 5, 2015, https://www.theguardian.com/news/datablog/2015/jun/05/french-more-holidays-work-less-productivity.

3. Justin McCarthy, "Six in 10 Americans Took a Vacation in 2017," Gallup, January 3, 2020, https://news.gallup.com/poll/224843/six-americans-took-vacation-2017.aspx.

4. Stephen Petterson, John M. Westfall, Benjamin Miller, "Projected Deaths of Despair During the Coronavirus Recession" (Oakland, CA: Well Being Trust, May 2020), https://wellbeingtrust.org/wp-content/uploads/2020/05/WBT_Deaths-of-Despair_COVID-19-FINAL-FINAL.pdf.

5. Julianne Holt-Lunstad and Timothy B. Smith, "Loneliness and Social Isolation as Risk Factors for Mortality: A Meta-Analytic Review," *All Faculty Publications* (Provo, UT: Brigham Young University, 2015), https://scholarsarchive.byu.edu/cgi/viewcontent.cgi?article=3024&context=facpub.

6. Thomas R. Insel, "Assessing the Economic Costs of Serious Mental Illness," *American Journal of Psychiatry* 165, no. 6 (June, 2008), https://ajp.psychiatry-online.org/doi/full/10.1176/appi.ajp.2008.08030366.

7. Jean M. Twenge et al., "Declines in Sexual Frequency among American Adults, 1989–2014," *Archives of Sexual Behavior* 46 (November 2017): 2389–2401, https://doi.org/10.1007/s10508-017-0953-1.

8. Twenge, "Declines in Sexual Frequency."

9. Tara Bahrampour, "Americans Are Having Less Sex than They Once Did," *Washington Post*, March 7, 2017, https://www.washingtonpost.com/local/social-issues/americans-having-less-sex-than-they-once-did/2017/03/06/e367ce58-0298-11e7-b9fa-ed727b644a0b_story.html.

10. "Body Image – Boys." MediaSmarts (website), August 22, 2014, https://mediasmarts.ca/body-image/body-image-boys.

11. Kristen R. Ghodsee, *Why Women Have Better Sex Under Socialism: And Other Arguments for Economic Independence* (New York: Bold Type Books, 2018).

12. Statista Research Department, "Number of Mobile Phone Users Worldwide 2015–2020," Statista (website), November 23, 2016, https://www.statista.com/statistics/274774/forecast-of-mobile-phone-users-worldwide/.

13. "Are You Addicted to Your Phone?" Asurion (website), March 2018, https://www.asurion.com/connect/tech-tips/are-you-addicted-to-your-phone/.

14. "How Does Nature Impact Our Wellbeing?," Taking Charge of Your Health & Wellbeing (website), University of Minnesota, accessed November 22, 2020, https://www.takingcharge.csh.umn.edu/how-does-nature-impact-our-wellbeing.

15. "How Does Nature?," University of Minnesota.

6. BODY. FULL. NESS.: NOT YOUR MOTHER'S MINDFULNESS

1. "Ecosystem," Wikimedia Foundation, accessed November 11, 2020, https://en.wikipedia.org/wiki/Ecosystem.

2. Bessel van der Kolk, *The Body Keeps the Score: Brain, Mind, and Body in the Healing of Trauma* (New York: Penguin, 2014).

3. Moira Gatens, "Power, Bodies and Difference," in *Feminist Theory and the Body: A Reader*, ed. Janet Price and Margrit Shildrick (New York: Routledge, 1999), 225–34. See also Christine Caldwell, "Mindfulness and Bodyfulness: A New Paradigm," *The Journal of Contemplative Inquiry* 1, no. 1 (2014): 90.

4. Tim Lomas, "Where Does the Word 'Mindfulness' Come From?" *Psychology Today*, March 16, 2016, https://www.psychologytoday.com/us/blog/mindfulness-wellbeing/201603/where-does-the-word-mindfulness-come.

5. Elisabeth Almekinder, "The N.E.A.T. Way to Exercise for a Longer, Healthier Life," Blue Zones (website), https://www.bluezones.com/2020/01/the-neat-way-to-exercise-for-a-longer-healthier-life/.

6. Gwen McHale, "The Power of Containment," *Somatic Therapy* (blog), April 4, 2016, https://gwenmchale.wordpress.com/2016/08/04/the-power-of-containment/.

7. Stephen Cope, *Yoga and the Quest for the True Self* (New York: Bantam, 2000).

8. "Ecstatic Living Institute of Tantra," *Ecstatic Living Institute* (blog), accessed November 22, 2020, https://www.ecstaticliving.com/blog.

9. Nayyirah Waheed, *Salt* (self-pub., CreateSpace, 2013).

10. Thomas F. Cash, "Body Image: Past, Present, and Future," *Body Image* 1, no. 1 (January 2004): 1–5, https://doi.org/10.1016/S1740-1445(03)00011-1.

11. Sonya Renee Taylor, *Your Body Is Not an Apology: The Power of Radical Self Love* (Oakland, CA: Berrett-Koehler Publishers, 2018).

7. OUR ISSUES ARE IN OUR TISSUES

1. Carl Jung, *The Archetypes and The Collective Unconscious* (Princeton, NJ: Princeton University Press, 1981).

2. Kerri Kelly, "Wellness Beyond Whiteness," CTZNWELL, May 20, 2020, https://www.ctznwell.org/ctznpodcast/wellness-beyond-whiteness.

3. Dan Heath, *Upstream: The Quest to Solve Problems Before They Happen* (New York: Avid Reader Press, 2020).

4. Jane Turner and Brian Kelly, "Emotional Dimensions of Chronic Disease," *Western Journal of Medicine* 172, no. 2 (February 2000): 124–28, https://www.ncbi.nlm.nih.gov/pmc/articles/PMC1070773/.

5. van der Kolk, *The Body Keeps the Score.*

6. Marilyn Van Derber, *Miss America by Day: Lessons Learned from Ultimate Betrayals and Unconditional Love* (Denver: Oak Hill Ridge Press, 2003).

7. Peter A. Levine and Ann Frederick, *Waking the Tiger: Healing Trauma* (Berkeley, CA: North Atlantic Books, 1997).

8. Leyla Roksan Caglar, "Traumatized Broca's Area: A Linguistic Analysis of Speech in Posttraumatic Stress Disorder" (master's thesis, Utrecht University, 2012), https://aphasia.talkbank.org/publications/2012/Caglar12.pdf.

9. David DeSteno, "The Kindness Cure," The *Atlantic*, July 21, 2015, https://www.theatlantic.com/health/archive/2015/07/mindfulness-meditation-empathy-compassion/398867. See also Gesa Kappen, Johan C. Karremans, William J. Burk, and Asuman Buyukcan-Tetik, "On the Association Between Mindfulness and Romantic Relationship Satisfaction: The Role of Partner Acceptance," *Mindfulness* 9, no. 5 (2018): 1543–56, https://www.ncbi.nlm.nih.gov/pmc/articles/PMC6153889/.

10. Norman Farb et al., "Interoception, Contemplative Practice, and Health," *Frontiers in Psychology* 6 (2015): 763. Sahib S. Khalsa, David Rudrauf, Antonio

R. Damasio, Richard J. Davidson, Antoine Lutz, and Daniel Tranel, "Interoceptive Awareness in Experienced Meditators," *Psychophysiology* 45, no. 4 (2008): 671–77.

11. A. D. Craig, "How Do You Feel—Now? The Anterior Insula and Human Awareness," *Nature Reviews Neuroscience* 10 (2009): 59–70, https://pubmed. ncbi.nlm.nih.gov/19096369/.

12. E. Martin, C. T. Dourish, P. Rotshtein, M. S. Spetter, and S. Higgs, "Interoception and Disordered Eating: A Systematic Review," *Neuroscience and Behavioral Reviews* 107 (2019): 166–91, https://doi:10.1016/j.neubiorev.2019.08.020.

13. Charles J. Wysocki and George Preti, "Facts, Fallacies, Fears, and Frustrations with Human Pheromones," *Anatomical Record* 281A, no. 1 (November 2004): 1201–11, https://doi.org/10.1002/ar.a.20125. See also J. Verhaeghe, R. Gheysen, and P. Enzlin, "Pheromones and Their Effect on Women's Mood and Sexuality," *Facts, Views & Vision in ObGyn* 5, no. 3 (2013): 189–95, https://www.ncbi.nlm.nih.gov/pmc/articles/PMC3987372/.

14. Asmir Gračanin, Lauren M. Bylsma, and Ad J. J. M. Vingerhoets, "Is Crying a Self-Soothing Behavior?" *Frontiers in Psychology* (May 28, 2014): https://www.ncbi.nlm.nih.gov/pmc/articles/PMC4035568/. See also Mandy Oaklander, "The Science of Crying," *Time*, March 16, 2016, https://time.com/4254089/science-crying/.

15. Weizmann Institute of Science, "Emotional Signals Are Chemically Encoded in Tears, Researchers Find," *ScienceDaily*, January 7, 2011, https://www.sciencedaily.com/releases/2011/01/110106144741.htm.

16. Wendy Suzuki, "The Brain-Changing Benefits of Exercise," TED, November 2017, https://www.ted.com/talks/wendy_suzuki_the_brain_changing_benefits_of_exercise.

17. Henry Emmons, *The Chemistry of Joy: Overcoming Depression through Western Science and Eastern Wisdom* (New York: Simon & Schuster, 2006), 94.

18. Levine, *Waking the Tiger*.

19. Paolo Tozzi, "Does Fascia Hold Memories?" *Journal of Bodywork and Movement Therapies* 18, no. 2 (April 1, 2014): 259–65, https://www.bodywork-movementtherapies.com/article/S1360-8592(13)00192-7/fulltext.

20. Page Seiffert, "The Emotional Core, aka the Psoas," Pilates Nosara, February 7, 2017, https://www.pilatesnosara.com/post/2017/02/07/the-emotional-core-aka-the-psoas.

21. Ambarish Vijayaraghava, Venkatesh Doreswamy, Omkar Subbaramajois Narasipur, Radhika Kunnavil, and Nandagudi Srinivasamurthy, "Effect of Yoga Practice on Levels of Inflammatory Markers After Moderate and Strenuous Exercise," *Journal of Clinical and Diagnostic Research* 9, no. 6 (June 2015): https://www.ncbi.nlm.nih.gov/pmc/articles/PMC4525504/. See also

Roderik J. S. Gerritsen and Guido P. H. Band, "Breath of Life: The Respiratory Vagal Stimulation Model of Contemplative Activity," *Frontiers in Human Neuroscience* 12 (2018): https://www.ncbi.nlm.nih.gov/pmc/articles/PMC6189422/.

22. Anupama Tyagi and Marc Cohen, "Yoga and Heart Rate Variability: A Comprehensive Review of the Literature," *International Journal of Yoga* 9, no. 2 (July–December 2016): 97–113, https://www.ncbi.nlm.nih.gov/pmc/articles/PMC4959333/.

23. Kishore Kumar Katuri, Ankineedu Babu Dasari, Sruthi Kurapati, Narayana Rao Vinnakota, Appaiah Chowdary Bollepalli, and Ravindranath Dhulipalla, "Association of Yoga Practice and Serum Cortisol Levels in Chronic Periodontitis Patients with Stress-Related Anxiety and Depression," *Journal of International Society of Preventive and Community Dentistry* 6, no. 1 (January–February 2016): 7–14, https://www.ncbi.nlm.nih.gov/pmc/articles/PMC4784068//.

24. Yoko Yoshikawa, "Everybody Upside-Down," *Yoga Journal*, August 28, 2007, https://www.yogajournal.com/practice/everybody-upside-down.

25. David Emerson, "Toward Becoming a Trauma-Sensitive Yoga Teacher" (manual privately given during training, 2009), 16.

26. Traci Pedersen, "Muscular Strength Tied to Brain Health," *Psych Central*, August 8, 2018, https://psychcentral.com/news/2018/04/21/muscular-strength-tied-to-brain-health/134797.html.

8. THE PLEASURE PRINCIPLE

1. Morten L. Kringelbach and Kent C Berridge, "The Neuroscience of Happiness and Pleasure," *Social Research* 77, no. 2 (2010): 659–678, https://www.ncbi.nlm.nih.gov/pmc/articles/PMC3008658/.

2. Kent C. Berridge and Morten L Kringelbach, "Pleasure Systems in the Brain," *Neuron* 86, no. 3 (2015): 646–64, https://doi.org/10.1016/j.neuron.2015.02.018.

3. Kringelbach and Berridge, "Neuroscience of Happiness."

4. Kringelbach and Berridge, "Neuroscience of Happiness."

5. Kringelbach and Berridge, "Neuroscience of Happiness."

6. Morten L. Kringelbach, *The Pleasure Center: Trust Your Animal Instincts* (New York: Oxford University Press, 2009).

7. Karen Doll, "23 Resilience Building Tools and Exercises," Positive Psychology (website), October 13, 2020, https://positivepsychology.com/resilience-activities-exercises/.

8. Sonya Taylor Brown, "Brené with Sonya Renee Taylor on *The Body Is Not an Apology*, September 16, 2020, in *Unlocking Us*, podcast, MP3 audio, 1:17:19, https://brenebrown.com/podcast/brene-with-sonya-renee-taylor-on-the-body-is-not-an-apology/.

9. Email from the United States Association for Body Psychotherapy.

10. See more at https://www.stephenporges.com/.

11. "Science of the Heart: Exploring the Role of the Heart in Human Performance," HeartMath Institute (website), https://www.heartmath.org/research/science-of-the-heart/heart-brain-communication/.

12. Adam Hadhazy, "Think Twice: How the Gut's 'Second Brain' Influences Mood and Well-Being," *Scientific American*, February 12, 2010, https://www.scientificamerican.com/article/gut-second-brain/.

13. "The Three Brains: Why Your Head, Heart, and Gut Sometimes Conflict," Australian Spinal Research Foundation, July 26, 2016, https://spinalresearch.com.au/three-brains-head-heart-gut-sometimes-conflict/.

14. Brian Gorman, "Change Leadership: Why Your Head, Heart, and Gut Are Critical to Listen To," *Forbes*, March 4, 2019, https://www.forbes.com/sites/forbescoachescouncil/2019/03/04/change-leadership-why-your-head-heart-and-gut-are-critical-to-listen-to/#681e14134a96. See also Vicky Karkou, Supritha Aithal, Ania Zubala, and Bonnie Meekums, "Effectiveness of Dance Movement Therapy in the Treatment of Adults with Depression," *Frontiers in Psychology* 10 (2019): https://doi.org/10.3389/fpsyg.2019.00936.

15. Bessel van der Kolk is quoted in this article by Eric Newhouse, "Vets Experiencing Trauma Can't Respond to Reason," *Psychology Today*, December 17, 2015, https://www.psychologytoday.com/us/blog/invisible-wounds/201512/vets-experiencing-trauma-cant-respond-reason.

9. MOTION IS LOTION

1. Dan Heath, *Upstream: The Quest to Solve Problems before They Happen* (New York: Simon & Schuster, 2020).

2. Sarah Otto-Combs, "An Ayurvedic Perspective on Sex, Libido, and How to Entice the Dosha Types," Siddha Labs, February 13, 2019, https://www.siddhalabs.com/blogs/all/an-ayurvedic-perspective-on-sex-libido-and-how-to-entice-the-dosha-types.

3. Julie Checknita, "Sex for Your Dosha: The 6 Ayurvedic Sexual Guidelines," *Elephant Journal*, December 15, 2019, https://www.elephantjournal.com/2019/12/sex-according-to-ayurveda/.

10. LEAVE YOUR MIND AND COME TO YOUR SENSES

1. Anette Kjellgren and Jessica Westman, "Beneficial Effects of Treatment with Sensory Isolation in Flotation-Tank as a Preventive Health-Care Intervention: A Randomized Controlled Pilot Trial," *BMC Complementary and Alternative Medicine* 14, no. 417 (2014), https://doi.org/10.1186/1472-6882-14-417.

2. "Theta Waves and Float Therapy," Serene Dreams (website), https://serenedreams.com/theta-waves-float-therapy/.

3. Valorie N. Salimpoor, Mitchel Benovoy, Kevin Larcher, Alain Dagher, and Robert J. Zatorre, "Anatomically Distinct Dopamine Release During Anticipation and Experience of Peak Emotion to Music," *Nature Neuroscience* 14 (2011): 257–262, http://www.nature.com/neuro/journal/v14/n2/abs/nn.2726.html.

4. Joanna Cazden, "Stalking the calm buzz: how the polyvagal theory links stage presence, mammal evolution, and the root of the vocal nerve," *Voice and Speech Review* 14, no. 2 (2020): 143–166, https://doi.org/10.1080/23268 263.2017.1390036.

5. Ralph Pawling, Peter R. Cannon, Francis P. McGlone, Susannah C. Walker, "C-Tactile Afferent Stimulating Touch Carries a Positive Affective Value," *PLoS ONE* 12, no. 3 (March 2017), https://doi.org/10.1371/journal.pone.0173457.

6. Shanely Pierce, "Touch Starvation Is a Consequence of COVID-19's Physical Distancing," TMC Health News, Texas Medical Center, May 15, 2020, https://www.tmc.edu/news/2020/05/touch-starvation/.

7. David Linden, *Touch: The Science of the Hand, Heart, and Mind* (New York: Penguin, 2016).

8. Blakeslee, "A Small Part of the Brain."

9. Blakeslee, "A Small Part of the Brain."

10. Quoted from Joseph Stromberg, "9 Surprising Facts about the Sense of Touch," *Vox*, January 28, 2015, https://www.vox.com/2015/1/28/7925737/touch-facts.

11. Jiageng Chen, Andrew Leber, Julie Golomb, "Attentional Capture Alters Feature Perception," *Journal of Experimental Psychology: Human Perception and Performance* 45, no. 11 (November 2019): 1443–1454, https://psycnet.apa.org/buy/2019-49303-001.

12. Saul L. Miller and Jon K. Maner, "Ovulation as a Male Mating Prime: Subtle Signs of Women's Fertility Influence Men's Mating Cognition and Behavior," *Journal of Personality and Social Psychology* 100, no. 2 (2011): 295–308, https://doi.org/10.1037/a0020930.

13. Simon M. McCrea, "Intuition, Insight, and the Right Hemisphere: Emergence of Higher Sociocognitive Functions," *Psychology Research and Behavior Management* 3 (2010): 1–39, https://doi.org/10.2147/prbm.s7935.

14. James Baldwin, *The Fire Next Time* (New York: Vintage, 1992), 43.

11. GIVE IT TO ME, GIVE IT TO ME

1. Christian C. Joyal, Amélie Cossette, Vanessa Lapierre, "What Exactly Is an Unusual Sexual Fantasy?" *Journal of Sexual Medicine* 12, no. 2 (February 2015): 328–340, https://doi.org/10.1111/jsm.12734.

2. Debby Herbenick et al., "Sexual Diversity in the United States: Results from a Nationally Representative Probability Sample of Adult Women and Men," *PloS ONE* 12, no. 7 (July 2017): doi:10.1371/journal.pone.0181198.

3. Emily Nagoski, *Come as You Are: The Surprising New Science That Will Transform Your Sex Life* (New York: Simon and Schuster, 2015).

4. Nicole Daedone, *Slow Sex: The Art and Craft of the Female Orgasm* (New York: Grand Central Life & Style, 2011).

5. David Huron and Elizabeth Hellmuth Margulis, "Musical Expectancy and Thrills," in *Handbook of Music and Emotion: Theory, Research, Applications*, eds. Patrik Juslin and John Sloboda (New York: Oxford University Press, 2011), 591.

6. Osmo Kontula and Anneli Miettinen, "Determinants of Female Sexual Orgasms," *Socioaffective Neuroscience & Psychology* 6, no. 31624 (2016): https://doi.org/10.3402/snp.v6.31624.

7. Kim Wallen and Elisabeth A. Lloyd, "Female Sexual Arousal: Genital Anatomy and Orgasm in Intercourse," *Hormones and Behavior* 59, no. 5 (2011): 780–92. https://doi.org/10.1016/j.yhbeh.2010.12.004.

8. Annette Bischof-Campbell, Peter Hilpert, Andrea Burri, Karoline Bischof, "Body Movement Is Associated with Orgasm during Vaginal Intercourse in Women," *Journal of Sex Research* 56, no. 3 (October 2018): 356–66, https://doi.org/10.1080/00224499.2018.1531367.

12. BE A HUMBLE WARRIOR

1. Steve Horsmon, "How to Avoid the Pursuer-Distancer Pattern in Your Relationship," The Gottman Institute, March 6, 2017, https://www.gottman.com/blog/how-to-avoid-the-pursuer-distancer-pattern-in-your-relationship/.

2. Diane Poole-Heller, *The Power of Attachment: How to Create Deep and Lasting Intimate Relationships* (Louisville, CO: Sounds True, 2019).

3. Alexandra Alter, "Erica Jong's 'Fear of Dying' Defies the Sunset of Sex," *New York Times*, September 7, 2015, Books, https://www.nytimes.com/2015/09/08/books/erica-jongs-fear-of-dying-defies-the-sunset-of-sex.html.

4. Alison Pereto, "Patients over 60? Screen for STIs," Athena Health (website), May 16, 2018, https://www.athenahealth.com/knowledge-hub/clinical-trends/over-60-stis-may-not-be-done-you.

5. Twenge, "Declines in Sexual Frequency."

6. D. Herbenick, V. Schick, S. A. Sanders, M. Reece, and J. D. Fortenberry, "Pain Experienced during Vaginal and Anal Intercourse among Male-Female Partners: Findings from a Nationally Representative Probability Study in the United States," *Journal of Sexual Medicine* 12, no. 4 (2015): 1040–51.

7. John Mordechai Gottman et al., "Observing Gay, Lesbian and Heterosexual Couples' Relationships: Mathematical Modeling of Conflict Interaction," *Journal of Homosexuality* 45, no. 1 (2003): 65–91, https://doi.org/10.1300/J082v45n01_04.

8. Jack Morin, *The Erotic Mind: Unlocking the Inner Sources of Passion and Fulfillment* (New York: Harper Perennial, 1996).

9. Simcha Shtull, "7 Verbs . . . Better Loving (E. Perel)," *The Relationship Blog*, May 15, 2018, http://www.therelationshipblog.net/2017/05/7-verbs-better-loving-e-perel/.

13. MAGNETIC INTIMACY

1. David Whyte, *Essentials* (Langley, WA: Many Rivers Press, 2020).
2. Stefanie Hanes, "Singles Nation: Why So Many Americans Are Unmarried," *Christian Science Monitor*, June 14, 2015, https://www.csmonitor.com/USA/Society/2015/0614/Singles-nation-Why-so-many-Americans-are-unmarried.
3. Laura Usher, "Conscious Sex: Surrendering to the Bliss of Sexual Energy as a Path to Healing and Growth," La Loba, blog, March 9, 2020, https://laloba.com.au/blogs/blog/conscious-sex-surrendering-to-the-bliss-of-sexual-energy-as-a-path-to-healing-and-growth.
4. Phillip Moffitt, "The Yoga of Relationships," *Yoga Journal*, updated April 5, 2017, https://www.yogajournal.com/yoga-101/the-yoga-of-relationships.
5. Shani Silver, "The Insanity of Being Single," *Medium*, Shani Silver, January 21, 2020, https://shanisilver.medium.com/the-insanity-of-being-single-b092d63e735a.
6. Patricia Love, *The Truth About Love: The Highs, the Lows, and How You Can Make It Last Forever* (New York: Fireside, 2001), 171.

14. EROTIC PLEASURE

1. Tuuli Kukkonen, "Still Going Strong: Sexuality in Older Adults," TedxGuelphU, March 20, 2017, 14:48, https://www.youtube.com/watch?v=pqLhP-POEJB4&lc=UgzL7qbChhCXQqlU7IZ4AaABAg&ab_channel=TEDxTalks.
2. For more on sexual satisfaction, see Raymond Rosen and Gloria Bachmann, "Sexual Well-Being, Happiness, and Satisfaction, in Women: The Case for a New Conceptual Paradigm," *Journal of Sex and Marital Therapy* 34, no. 4 (2008): 291–97, https://doi.org/10.1080/00926230802096234. See also David Lee, Bram Vanhoutte, James Nazroo, and Neil Pendleton, "Sexual Health and Positive Subjective Well-Being in Partnered Older Men and Women," *The Journals of Gerontology, Series B, Psychological Sciences, and Social Sciences* 71, no. 4 (2016): 698–710, https://doi.org/10.1093/geronb/gbw018.
3. Rosen and Bachmann, "Sexual Well-Being."
4. Nagoski, *Come As You Are.*
5. Jack Morin, *The Erotic Mind.*
6. Ashlyn Brady et al., "Gratitude Increases the Motivation to Fulfill a Partner's Sexual Needs," *Social Psychological and Personality Science* (April 2020), https://journals.sagepub.com/doi/abs/10.1177/1948550619898971
7. Paul Bloom, *How Pleasure Works: The New Science of Why We Like What We Like* (New York: W. W. Norton, 2011).

8. Gary Chapman, *The 5 Love Languages: The Secret to Love That Lasts* (Chicago: Northfield Publishing, 2015).

9. See more at https://missjaiya.com/.

10. Jessie Lucier, "We Asked: Do Yogis Have Better Sex?" *Yoga Journal*, updated April 13, 2017, https://www.yogajournal.com/lifestyle/asked-yogis-better-sex.

11. Vikas Dhikav et al., "Yoga in Female Sexual Functions," *The Journal of Sexual Medicine* 7, no. 2 (February 2010): 964–970, https://www.sciencedirect.com/science/article/abs/pii/S1743609515329143.

12. Wednesday Martin, "The Bored Sex," *The Atlantic*, February 14, 2019, https://www.theatlantic.com/ideas/archive/2019/02/women-get-bored-sex-long-term-relationships/582736/.

13. Brady, "Gratitude Increases the Motivation."

14. Audre Lorde, *The Uses of the Erotic: The Erotic as Power* (Tucson, AZ: Kore Press, 1978).

APPENDIX

1. Lena Schmidt, "Find the Balance between Your Feminine and Masculine Energy," Chopra (website), May 31, 2019, https://chopra.com/articles/find-the-balance-between-your-feminine-and-masculine-energy.

2. Anodea Judith, *Eastern Body, Western Mind: Psychology and the Chakra System as a Path to the Self* (New York: Celestial Arts, 2004).

3. Geneen Roth, *Women, Food and God: An Unexpected Path to Almost Everything* (New York: Scribner, 2016).

Index

creativity
play and, 31, 32–33
sex and, 227–28

Daedone, Nicole, 198
Darwin, Charles, 138
dating, 234–36
Descartes, René, 51
desire
body memory and, 190–91
differences in, 240–42
feeling deserving of, 184–88
learning what we want, 192–95
maintaining, 242–50
self-pleasuring and, 195–97
self-worth and, 188–89
See also sexual and erotic pleasure
differentiation, 216–17
discernment, 145–46
disconnection, 2
as dissociation, 118, 169
technology and, 80–81, 82–84
See also mind-body disconnection
disembodiment, 46–47, 159
trauma and, 121
distancer-pursuer dynamic, 214–16
doshas, 148–49, 153–55, 266–69
Doyle, Glennon, 65

Einstein, Albert, 156, 181
embodied mindfulness, 20, 102,
124–29. *See also* bodyfulness
Emerson, David, 106, 135
Emmons, Henry, 132
emotional body memory, 122–23
emotional intimacy, 217–19
emotional touch system, 177
emotions
mind-body split and, 51–52
releasing, 107, 109–10
tending and befriending, 88–90

energetic boundaries, 156–57
epicurean lifestyle, 92–94
epigenetics, 120–21
erogenous zones, 177, 197–98
erotic energy, 226–27. *See also* sexual
and erotic pleasure
erotic languages, 248
erotic polarity, 247
essence, unchanging, 74–75
eye gazing, 246

fight-flight-freeze response, 118–19,
140, 190, 215, 241
Fisher, Dr. Helen, 138
flirting, 236–37
flow channel, 34, 35, 119
FOMO (fear of missing out), 72, 91
Forbes, Bo, 159
foreplay, 31, 32, 227–28
syncing, 249–50
Frankl, Viktor, 104
Freud, Sigmund, 50–51

gender fluidity, 73–74
gender identity, 191
differences in, 64–66
sexual violence and, 67
as social construct, 61–63
Ghodsee, Kristen, 82
grief, 209
reunion, 237–38
gut (enteric) brain, 142

Hanson, Rick, 119
happiness, pleasure and, 25–26,
27, 139
Hatfield, Elaine, 67
heart (cardiac) brain, 142
Hebb, Donald, 145
Heller, Diane Poole, 216
Hippocrates, 54

holistic medicine, 53–54

How to Change Your Mind (Pollan), 54

Humble Warrior pose, 210–11

inner wisdom, bodyfulness and, 112–13

interoception, 102, 127–29, 146

intimacy, 1, 206–7

  attachment styles and, 212–16

  differentiation and, 216–17

  physical and emotional, 217–19

  risk management and, 208–10

  strength and, 210–12

  See also relationships

intuition, 180–81

JOMO (joy of missing out), 91–92

Jong, Erica, 219

joy

  foreboding, 40

  pleasure and, 3–4, 25–26, 27

Jung, Carl, 31, 121

Kierkegaard, Søren, 159

Kotler, Steven, 34

Kritzer, Wendy, 122

Lamott, Anne, 93

language, trauma and, 124–25

Lao Tzu, 209

Levine, Peter, 122–23

Ley, David, 49

LGBTTQQIAAP community, 205

Linden, David, 176, 177

lively pleasure, 27, 33–36, 216, 256

Love, Pat, 237–38

Lowen, Alexander, 159

magnetism, 236–37

Maslow, Abraham, 155

masturbation, 195–97

Mc Hale, Gwen, 109–10

McDowell, Emily, 74–75

medicine, conventional

  holistic medicine vs., 53–54

  mind-body split and, 45, 49–52, 124

meditation, 15, 20–21, 127

memory retrieval, trauma and, 125–26

mental health/psychology

  early views of women, 50–51

  interoception and, 129

  mind-body split and, 5, 117

#MeToo movement, 67

Michael Pollan, 54

mind-body disconnection, 5, 15, 46–48

  body as machine and, 51–54

  conventional medicine and, 45, 49–52, 124

  repression and, 48–49

mindfulness, 5, 6, 102

  limitations of, 126–27

  See also embodied mindfulness

Mischke-Reeds, Manuela, 29

Moffitt, Phillip, 233–34

Morin, Jack, 222

movement activities, 72–73, 144

  communal, 143–44

  for discharging and releasing, 107–11

  as medicine, 129–35

  neuroscience and, 131–32

movement therapies, 18, 134–35

Nagoski, Emily, 241

nature deficit disorder, 72–73, 83

needs, hierarchy of, 155

negativity bias, 119

nervous system

  as conductor, 118–21

  regulation and, 123–24, 141–42

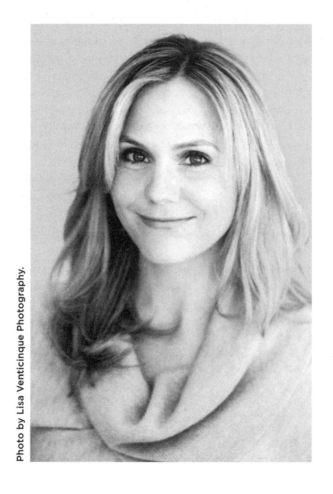

About the Author

Rachel Allyn, PhD, is a licensed psychologist, certified yoga instructor, and retreat leader. She is the founder of YogaPsych, PLLC, a psychotherapy practice for adults that blends Western medicine with Eastern philosophy and connects the mind with the body. She has been in private practice for fifteen years working with individuals and couples dealing with relationships, intimacy, sexual health, life transitions, depression, and anxiety.

As a child raised in Minnesota, she was drawn to all kinds of outdoor activities, later realizing that movement was her medicine to keep her focused and resilient. She left the Midwest to get her BA from Williams College in Massachusetts. Then she promptly did what any plucky graduate of a liberal arts school might do: parlayed her political science degree into work as a reporter for a San Francisco television station. Logic aside, this led her to graduate school in psychology to satiate her curiosity about why humans do what they do and how they can feel more connected and joyful. After getting a PhD from the California School of Professional Psychology in San Francisco, she became certified as a yoga instructor and later completed additional trainings in trauma-informed yoga.

She helps clients develop a bodyfulness practice, which builds from mindfulness to more dynamically engage the body's wisdom and is based on research that past trauma can get stuck in the body unless we have safe ways to discharge it.

Dr. Allyn has spoken nationally at conferences, led workshops and seminars in a multitude of settings, and delivered a TEDx talk in 2019 on reconnecting to the body to reclaim pleasure. She also facilitates wellness retreats throughout the world.

From 2016 to 2019, Dr. Allyn wrote a monthly advice column called "Ask Dr. Rachel." She's been quoted in books and magazines including *Yoga Journal, Women's Health, Outside, Good Housekeeping,* and *Cosmopolitan* and has been featured on many podcasts.

Her ultimate message is that even in this often challenging world, connection to life's pleasures remains right there inside of you. When not spreading this message, she divides her time between her travels, the trails, and anyplace she can sing karaoke.